INTELLIGENT FITNESS

T0043537

'Results come not just from working hard, but from working smart. With Simon's help, I've been able to sustain the highest level of health and fitness through several action movie franchises without injury or misery. I am one of countless others within the entertainment industry who trust him completely. It's thrilling that Simon's proven strategies will now be available to all.'
BRYCE DALLAS HOWARD

'Simon is extremely rigorous and diligent: always prepared and punctual. He is unfailingly respectful, careful and kind. He knows when to work hard: he knows when to push a little further, to encourage you out of your comfort zone. He taught me so much.'
TOM HIDDLESTON

'If you had told me I'd be in the best shape of my life at forty-one, I would have said you were crazy. Simon was able to achieve that by not only changing my workout regimen, but by changing my entire mental approach to the whole process. Normally getting in shape for anything feels like a one-shot deal. Go hard, hit a number, celebrate, go back to old habits. But working with Simon is a completely holistic experience. In his mind, the end result is just a step of a longer journey. From diet and cardio to heavy lifts and recovery treatments, Simon takes great care to push your body in incremental steps rather than vicious shifts in weight or appearance ... He makes you see and appreciate for yourself the massive difference between getting in shape and getting healthy.'
JOHN KRASINSKI

'Simon, working with you has always been a great pleasure. Not only are you the best trainer but you are also the funniest. You always make me laugh so much and, for the abs, there is nothing better!' **LÉA SEYDOUX**

INTELLIGENT FITNESS

The Smart Way To Reboot Your Body And Get In Shape

SIMON WATERSON

With a foreword by
DANIEL CRAIG

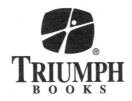

TRIUMPH
B O O K S

FOREWORD BY DANIEL CRAIG

Without Simon's help and guidance, I wouldn't have made it through fifteen years of playing James Bond. From 5 a.m. call times on wet and windy sets at Pinewood Studios to twelve-hour night shoots hanging precariously off the back of some moving vehicle and in exotic locations around the world, Simon was always right by my side.

Bond takes a battering – which he should, as a secret agent – and Simon was always there, always helping and supporting. He'd prepare me and, when necessary, repair me too when some knee or elbow joint gave out. Simon put in endless hours of rehab and treatment after the inevitable injuries. For all five of my Bond films, he was also always alongside me in the gym, a training partner as well as a trainer, doing every single exercise that he had asked me to do. Simon understood what I was going through to get in shape for Bond because he was experiencing just the same beside me.

Simon's curiosity, his commitment, humility and willingness to learn are what make him such a unique and talented trainer. You're in rare air when you're making a Bond movie, and the first time that Simon and I went out for dinner, we spoke about how I wanted the character to look and move. Simon, who took notes that evening, says that I used the word 'imposing'.

To play Bond, you need a lot of energy – you have to bring an intensity to the long days and nights, with the shoots lasting for months – and I couldn't have been in better hands with Simon, who had trained Pierce Brosnan for a couple of Bond movies before me. I was in my thirties when I shot my first Bond film, *Casino Royale*, and in my fifties for my fifth, *No Time to Die*, and every time Simon ensured – by starting slowly and building up to pre-production boot camps – that I had the conditioning I needed to portray Bond.

While Simon gave me a little longer to prepare for *No Time to Die* than I had for my previous Bond movies – it took around a year – we were both still just as competitive and ambitious as we had been for *Casino Royale* and the other three films. We weren't going to use age as an excuse for lowering our standards. In fact, on the first day of the main shoot, I believe I was as fit as I had ever been.

For every Bond film, I wanted to do as much of the stunt work as I could, and that was possible because of Simon's intelligent approach to fitness, and the way he put as much focus on my recovery and nutrition as he did on my training. It's been an honour to have worked with him.

INTRODUCTION

LOOK, MOVE, FEEL, SLEEP
AND RECOVER LIKE A FILM STAR

From *Jurassic World* and Indiana Jones to *The Avengers* and *The Fast and the Furious*, I have been turning actors into athletes for more than twenty-five years. As a health and fitness coach in the film industry, I work with actors to enable them to portray some of cinema's most iconic and athletic characters.

Using my 'intelligent fitness' approach, I've been fortunate enough to have trained actors for some major movie transformations. I prepared Daniel Craig for all five of his James Bond films, starting with *Casino Royale* right through to *No Time to Die*. I transformed Chris Evans for *Captain America*, one of the first films in the Marvel Cinematic Universe, my task being to turn a superhero from the pages of a comic book into human form. I also worked with Chris Pratt on the first *Guardians of the Galaxy* film, another Marvel production with a key aesthetic shot focusing on an actor's physique. On the Star Wars set, the joke was that the franchise should have been renamed 'Spa Wars' after so many of the cast got into the training and wellness that my team and I were offering.

I wouldn't be doing this job if I hadn't first been a marine commando for seven years. It was in the military – where your team or unit is only ever as strong as the weakest member – that

I discovered just how much I enjoyed helping others to improve and achieve their fitness goals. That feeling has stayed with me through my career as a fitness coach – it's so satisfying to help actors to do their jobs well on screen, and to also improve their health and wellbeing for life. It's even more rewarding than reaching my own fitness objectives.

After leaving the military, I became a trainer and started writing for fitness magazines, which is how I came to the attention of the James Bond producers. The first production that I was engaged on was a Bond film, working with Pierce Brosnan on *The World is Not Enough* in the late 1990s.

The physical expectations placed on actors are now greater than ever before. Certainly, it is a very different industry to the one I experienced when training Pierce. Back then, fitness was on the periphery of the film industry – now it's central to most productions I work on, especially the big action movies, such as Bond and the Marvel franchise. It's no longer just a case of actors turning up and performing. As well as delivering their lines and hitting their marks, they're expected to portray the right look while maintaining fitness and conditioning throughout the shoot.

Unfortunately, you can't act fit; there are no special effects that can help you there. That's why studios contact me – to take responsibility for the health and wellbeing of these actors to get them through a long shoot without injury or illness. I'm there to enable the actors to do their jobs effectively and safely. As an actor, if you're out of action for a couple of weeks or even longer, that's potentially very costly for a studio.

Until now, I have been fairly low-key about the projects I have worked on. But here, for the first time, and with the active encouragement of many of the A-list actors I have worked with, I'm going to be sharing my highly effective methods. I hope that my intelligent fitness approach will help you to achieve your own fitness goals.

FROM BASIC TO BOND

This is by no means an intimidating fitness manual aimed at the super advanced. The purpose of this book is to create a highly accessible and practical guide for everyone – men and women of all levels and abilities. Physical and mental wellbeing shouldn't just be for film stars on set. Over the following chapters, I want to provide you with all the guidance and encouragement that you'll need to enjoy sustainable health and fitness in your own life.

As the audience, we sit in a cinema with our popcorn, being entertained for a couple of hours. You might not realize how many months of discipline and dedication go into becoming James Bond and achieving the physical demands of the role alongside portraying the character and telling a story. You can't play the part effectively without hard graft. But the same workout methods I've used with Daniel Craig for fifteen years can be practised by anyone, whether you're at a basic level of fitness or about to shoot a movie. My hope for you is that, by understanding the effective training programmes that are responsible for transforming actors into athletes, you will be motivated to reboot your own fitness.

To help you achieve your goals, and also to give you an unprecedented insight into fitness in the film world, I'm sharing the actual workouts I designed for my clients. From Blake Lively to Bryce Dallas Howard and from Benedict Cumberbatch to John Krasinski, I'll explain exactly how I guided these stars to peak fitness. You can choose whether to train like Daniel Craig did for *No Time to Die*, or follow the programme I created for his co-star, Léa Seydoux. Alternatively, you may be more interested in the workout I developed for Tom Hiddleston for *Kong* or those I devised for John Boyega and Adam Driver for two Star Wars movies, *The Last Jedi* and *The Rise of Skywalker* (though you might not ever swing a lightsabre in a fight, you'll have similar conditioning). What I hope you'll take from this book are the methods and tricks that I've found so effective with my clients, which will allow you to begin your own fitness journey or continue to build on what you may have already started.

My clients are all ages and abilities – age and current fitness level are no barrier to what you can achieve. I discovered this first-hand when I prepared Harrison Ford – who was in his late seventies – before he shot the fifth Indiana Jones film, forty years after the release of the iconic *Raiders of the Lost Ark*.

GET INSPIRED

People are always asking me whether they could ever really look like James Bond, a Bond girl or Captain America. The answer is that it's possible as long as you're dedicated, you follow my advice and you have the genetic capacity. But instead of trying to achieve a movie-star physique, and to become a version of what you see on screen, you might find it's more beneficial to use these transformations as inspiration to become the greatest possible version of yourself. I would like my stories, insights and anecdotes to motivate you to enhance your health and wellbeing, including boosting your energy, sleep and confidence.

Over the last twenty-five years, I've had some amazing experiences in the film world. I've worked with some incredible people in some extraordinary places and in some surreal situations, such as wandering around Soho in central London just after 5 a.m. with Benicio Del Toro, banging on the doors of coffee bars to get them to open up early for a post-workout espresso. Or 3.30 a.m. training sessions in the desert with Jake Gyllenhaal, racing against Benedict Cumberbatch over 100 metres (and losing) and playing table tennis with Adam Driver (and losing). I vividly remember the happiness on Bryce Dallas Howard's face when she mastered how to stand on one leg on a BOSU ball – a very wobbly piece of kit – with her eyes closed, when I was preparing her for running in high heels while escaping from dinosaurs in *Jurassic World*.

I also had a very unusual morning in a hotel gym in West

London when I trained Jake Gyllenhaal, Emily Blunt and Daniel Craig, one after another. Jake was my 9 a.m., followed by Emily at 10 a.m. and Daniel at 11 a.m. (it was like a red-carpet event). From Ralph Fiennes to Woody Harrelson, I've been fortunate enough to have worked with some of the most amazing actors in cinema today, who time and again have shown great commitment and focus to the programmes I have designed for them. When I trained Alden Ehrenreich to play Han Solo in *Solo: A Star Wars Story*, he was trying to emulate Harrison Ford's physicality – while it's tough to look like someone else, Alden was completely dedicated.

TRAINING 007

Bond has been a massive part of my professional life. I've been James Bond's personal trainer for more than twenty years during seven movies, from *The World is Not Enough* through to *No Time to Die*. As both a Bond fan and a health and fitness coach, it has been a privilege to have trained Pierce Brosnan for two films and then to have worked with Daniel Craig to help him achieve the physicality needed to play 007 for five movies, while also maintaining his energy and mental wellbeing. After all this time, including training numerous Bond girls, I've been made to feel part of the Bond family.

The first time I met Daniel, which was just days after he had been announced as the new Bond in October 2005, he had a bacon sandwich in one hand and a roll-up cigarette in the other. He was on the set of another production in Washington DC and I had flown out there after Barbara Broccoli, the producer of the James Bond series, called me to say that she had someone she wanted me to meet (when Barbara calls, you pick up). I was amused by the sight of Daniel holding his sandwich and roll-up. In that moment, I also knew I was going to have to get rid of some old habits and create some new ones. 'You must be the trainer,' Daniel said, to which I replied, 'Yes, and it starts right here.'

The transformation into James Bond, which took around a year for each movie, puts demands on an actor like no other role. He's the most iconic character in cinema, and playing the secret agent is also probably one of the most challenging roles – physically and mentally – that any actor will ever undertake. Becoming Bond means becoming an athlete, both on and off screen. On the evening of the day that we first met, Daniel and I went out for steaks and beers. He spoke about how he wanted the character to look and move, and the key word he used was 'imposing'. That's when we came up with a plan. I made some notes over dinner and went away to design a programme for him.

From that first meal together, I was very aware of what Daniel was willing to do to become Bond. Like the character, Daniel was relentless. He always showed up, day after day, without complaints or excuses. He had to trust in my plan – he put his health and wellbeing, and the physicality he wanted to bring to the screen, in my hands.

We were meticulous from the start. If there was ever the slightest chance that doing something extra would improve Daniel's athletic performance by just 1 per cent, we would do it. His attention to detail was extraordinary – when he was carrying a gun, for instance, he wanted his forearms to look as though he had been handling that weapon forever. We would take things to the next level, particularly during the pre-production boot camp in the final weeks of preparation, when we would train with the intensity of a boxer before a big fight.

Years after the movie's cinematic release, people still talk to me about that iconic beach scene in *Casino Royale*, when Daniel emerges from the ocean looking like a true action hero. Bond had never had such a powerful presence before. For me, an even more impactful episode in that same film was when he was tied to a seatless chair and tortured with a knotted rope by Le Chiffre, played by Mads Mikkelsen. We prepared for that scene to create an authentic aesthetic that was strong and raw. Even then, there was still something imposing, almost shocking, about Daniel on screen, which was exactly what we had talked about during dinner in Washington DC.

Daniel and I would work hard all week and then celebrate at the end, so an alternative title for this book could have been *Blood, Sweat and Beers*, because that's what it took off screen to get him to where he needed to be. But please don't be intimidated – as I'll explain in the chapters that follow, everyone can work out like Bond today, even if you're at the beginning of your fitness journey and have been living a sedentary existence on the sofa.

When I'm training a Bond girl, I'm always conscious not to compromise the actor's femininity through fitness. While she has to keep up with Bond – she might suddenly have to sprint, pick up a weapon or jump out of a plane – as a trainer you need her to have sleek, smooth and seamless movements. Everything needs to look completely effortless on screen. That was my theory when preparing Léa Seydoux for *Spectre* and *No Time to Die*.

There's no stereotypical Bond girl, but what they have in common is their elegance and finesse, the way they walk and the way they carry themselves. I've worked with several other Bond girls, including Eva Green, Halle Berry, Rosamund Pike, Gemma Arterton, Bérénice Marlohe and Olga Kurylenko. With the information and insights in this book, you can tap into my experiences and train like a Bond girl, too.

PERFORMANCE, NOT AESTHETIC

I want you to create your own bespoke fitness programme – one that's tailored just for you. Pick and choose what works, and create a personal exercise plan that will help you to achieve your fitness goals. You might find that some of the workouts in this book are suitable for where you're at right now, and there may be other bits that you don't like so much or that don't align with your objectives – and that's absolutely fine. As long as exercise is enjoyable and sustainable, and contains all the key elements to allow you to attain your goals, there's no wrong or right approach.

One of the key lessons I want to share with you in this book, which has become my mantra with many of my clients, is that you should be training for pure performance rather than aesthetic – and this is because aesthetic is a by-product of performance. The primary goal with actors in training is always to complete any production while maintaining energy and performance, and limiting illnesses and injuries. If you don't have performance as an actor, you won't survive some of the most demanding shooting schedules, which can last for more than six months, with stunts, action sequences and twelve-hour days. Muscles alone won't take you where you need to be.

To play the role of Bond successfully, Daniel had to convince audiences that he was capable of hurting people. Daniel once said to me that when he took his shirt off, he wanted to look as though he could do the job he was portraying; he needed that developed muscularity and air of menace. I love the in-depth sense of character and how his physique helped to give particular scenes their power. Our aim was to match the physicality to the character's mentality – strong, efficient and capable.

But in the role of James Bond, looks certainly aren't enough. To make a Bond film, you need athleticism to survive a shoot. You must have speed and agility for the stunt sequences, such as the scene in *No Time to Die* when Bond throws himself off the side of a bridge. The expectations on Daniel were immense during this final film, as indeed they had been for every Bond outing before that. You might be playing a secret agent, but there's no place to hide as Bond on set. You must be able to turn your athleticism on and off very quickly, working with time constraints because of the hours of natural light and factors arising from the cast and crew's general fatigue.

In the modern world, we are so consumed with physical appearance that we forget about the athletic performance and the way we need to feel to achieve this. Yet it has so many knock-on effects for how you can handle day-to-day life, and I believe fitness and wellbeing are absolutely key to getting the most out of every day.

FITNESS IS A FEELING

You probably picked up this book thinking about how you want to look. But have you spent any time considering how you want to feel? Everyone's always saying, 'I want to look like this.' But I believe what you should be saying is, 'I want to feel like this.' Once you have that self-awareness, the by-product is going to be the visual. Fitness isn't about achieving a particular look or image. Fitness is primarily about feelings. Whatever your goals, I'm going to help you to feel like a film star. And if you feel good on the inside, that's going to be reflected on the outside.

Before every workout, you need to have an honest conversation with yourself. I'll help you to ask the right questions, with the answers determining how intensely you train that day, or even whether you walk away and don't train at all, and perhaps do a recovery session instead.

I believe you won't achieve your goals if you're pushing yourself too hard, risking injury, illness and mental fatigue. You can be too extreme, and I often talk about this with my clients. Sometimes less is more. I'll explain how you can rest your brain, and even activate it or warm it up, just like any other muscle. That's why I've dedicated a chapter in this book to why you shouldn't give yourself a hard time, which was particularly relevant when I was training Adam Driver for Star Wars. I had to tell Adam when to slow down, and when it was more important to recover for progression rather than train for progression, as fatigue is your worst enemy and can lead to potential burnout.

Your brain might tell your body to stop – but it won't ever be the other way around. I think that part of my role is to monitor actors' moods as well as their physical conditioning. Working out should enhance and focus your mind. Your programme should boost your energy and give you a zest for life.

As with anything, you need to have a plan for your fitness and to know what your goals are, but it's crucial that you don't aim too high in the beginning. I believe you should have small goals that allow you to achieve incremental gains and experience a sense of progression. Start slowly: my clients always do.

If your fitness programme is going to be sustainable, you must have the right mindset and I'll share with you my belief that you should train like a child – it's about reigniting the simple joy and euphoria that you used to feel when you were young. Like riding your bike, throwing a rugby ball around, going for a swim or doing a mini triathlon with a friend. Avoiding boredom and stagnation is key, which is why I'll be encouraging you to have plenty of variety in your workouts. You should also be leaving your comfort zone and trying new things, or going back to what you used to enjoy.

STRENGTH AND WELLBEING IN RECOVERY

While you should train like a child, you ought to recover like a granddad – carefully, methodically and often slowly. Recovery is the most important element of your programme and should be scheduled like a training session. I'll be teaching you how to stimulate your body's natural healing processes to help speed up your recovery, allowing you to maintain your training week on week.

Sleep tends to be the best guide to how the rest of your fitness programme is going, and I'll help you to improve the quality of your sleep so that you become a 'performance sleeper'. You might be pleased to hear that this will also involve the benefits of dozing for twenty minutes a day, which I like to call an athlete's nap!

Injuries are inevitable for an actor on set and it's important to know how to manage them. Often, the greatest challenge is how to deal with the mental side of setbacks, and how to prevent yourself from slipping into a dark place (as I found out while writing this book, when I broke my ankle and required an operation). I'll share my experience of how to avoid losing faith in your fitness. Fitness is one of the only industries in which failure is a positive. It's time to embrace failure if you want to make real gains.

I'll also give you some advice on how to train more efficiently, and how to make sure you don't become completely reliant on gyms and complicated machines, and why you should be able to do your workout anywhere, as all you'll need is your own body and a theory or method. I'll introduce you to the incredibly effective 5–2 method, which I use regularly with my clients and consider to be the Holy Grail of fitness.

In the third part of this book, I'll be passing on the same tips and tricks about nutrition that I give actors, including the psychology behind eating six meals a day and how having daily shots of turmeric, ginger or wheatgrass can be useful for gut health as well as acting as an anti-inflammatory. I'll even include the recipe for the performance shake that Daniel and I would drink after a workout, as we walked from my gym at Pinewood Studios to the 007 stage.

When you embark on your fitness journey, it's really important that you don't take an extreme approach to nutrition, even though it can feel like such a good idea when you want to make big changes to how you look and feel. I believe that going on a diet is the biggest mistake you can make – it can potentially destroy your muscle tissue and metabolism as well as your mental wellbeing. It's far more sustainable to give yourself parameters, with theme days throughout the week, such as Vegetarian Mondays, Pescatarian Tuesdays and Red Meat Fridays.

Although the actors featured throughout these pages are great examples of my tried-and-tested methods, this book isn't about them. It's about you and how I can help you to achieve your fitness goals. Remember, this book is a toolbox. Pick and choose what works for you. Get inspired and then get to work, creating your own fitness programme. You'll be fitter than ever before, you'll have more energy and confidence, and you'll be sleeping better.

ESSENTIAL KIT

If you're going to be working out at home or don't have access to a gym, I would suggest investing in these five bits of kit, which are all relatively inexpensive and will play a key role in some of the exercises I will share with you later in the book.

BOSU BALL: I use this a lot in the workouts I design for my clients – it introduces instability, which means you have to create stability. BOSUs can be used either way up and are great for improving your balance and core strength.

AB ROLLER: This is a really useful piece of kit for working on your abdominal muscles (you will need one for Daniel Craig's *No Time to Die* workout).

SET OF EXERCISE BANDS: These are extremely versatile and can easily be used at home or in the park. It's a good idea to have at least three in a range of light, medium and heavy resistance, as different muscle groups require different levels of resistance.

DUMBBELLS: These have two uses – they add resistance to a number of key exercises, and you can also put them on the ground and use them as push-up handles, which will help with building strength when doing push-ups.

KETTLEBELLS: These are cast-iron weights with a handle on top for easy gripping. They're an excellent way of adding diversity and resistance to a number of exercises.

PART 1
TRAINING

1 | THINK BIG, BUT SET SMALL GOALS

Daniel Craig and I are both extremely competitive. We decided during the preparations for *No Time to Die* that we would try to turn him into the fittest fifty-year-old on the planet. Now that's a major fitness goal – about as ambitious as can be – so we broke that down into smaller or micro goals. Getting Daniel ready for *No Time to Die* took more than a year, and every week we would set modest objectives to aim for. For that film, as well as for the previous four Bond movies that I had trained Daniel for, we started slowly, and incrementally increased his fitness. It doesn't matter who you are or what condition you're in, there is no better motivation than hitting your small targets and feeling a sense of progression. By the end of pre-production for *No Time to Die*, we had achieved our primary goal: I can't imagine there being a fitter fifty-year-old in the world than Daniel at that time.

Ambition is important, but you need to know how to set your own achievable goals to ensure you're more likely to reach them, and possibly even exceed them. You can think big, but at the same time create a sustainable programme that enables you to attain your long-term objectives by taking small steps. The progression and sense of accomplishment you'll feel from hitting your mini targets is a great motivator and will carry you forward to potentially reach unprecedented levels of fitness and wellbeing.

In this chapter, I'm going to be sharing some insider tips and tricks on how to set your goals and start rebooting your personal fitness.

CLARITY IS KEY

While I was training Chris Evans for *Captain America*, we were always working towards a particular date. That was the day when they would shoot the 'reveal', in which Chris emerges from a pod after his transformation from Skinny Steve Rogers to Captain America. That date wasn't flexible as sets were being built and schedules had been made; I circled it on the calendar and it was etched in both of our minds.

In the same way, I think it can be helpful for you to have a clear goal to work towards, as I have always found that's what motivates most people. Ask yourself what you want. What are you looking to achieve with your own programme? Before you start creating your fitness regimen, you must first learn to explore what your personal objectives are, and be clear in your mind about the journey on which you're about to embark.

As a former marine, I recognize the importance of developing a structured plan, and part of that is having a date on which to focus. Mark your date on a calendar. You might be sedentary and just starting out on your fitness journey, or maybe you're already at an advanced level but looking to push yourself further. Either way, specifically set out where you want to be and when.

MAKING IT RELEVANT

While the core of Daniel's programme remained the same for each of his five Bond movies, there were subtle differences from film to film, reflecting relevance and age. Daniel was always conscious that the character and his physique should be evolving, and so the athleticism depicted in his first Bond outing, *Casino Royale*, was very different to that in his fifth, *No Time to Die*.

For *Casino Royale*, the character was very imposing. Daniel was physically bigger than he would be in the subsequent films, which was a conscious decision. For the second Bond movie, *Quantum of Solace*, we decided to drop a few pounds of muscle mass and gain speed, efficiency and agility. The suits he wore for that film were a bit more tailored and a little sleeker than they had been for *Casino Royale*. This theme continued throughout *Skyfall* and *Spectre*. In all of Daniel's Bond films there were 'aesthetic shots', with the camera focusing on his physique.

But, as with all the programmes I create for actors, the training was primarily about performance. We adjusted Daniel's training for each Bond movie to ensure it tied in to the script, as each would have differently choreographed fight scenes as well as other athletic sequences, such as sprinting, hurdling, falling and reacting, all of which I would condition and prepare him for. When I plan Daniel's programme for a film, I have to make sure every element is relevant to the movie. At the beginning of a Bond movie, there's always an athletic chase sequence, so he's going to need to sprint and move. As big and imposing as Daniel was for *Casino Royale*, I had to be careful that we didn't compromise on flexibility or dynamic movement.

Daniel always needed explosive movement. But everything he did – sprinting, hurdling obstacles, crashing through walls, picking something up off the floor, dropping down off buildings and jumping into moving cars – had to look effortless on screen. We did the conditioning for the stunts in the gym. Then he went from the gym to the stunt room to put this into practice, before going to the stage for filming.

With every film project, the workouts have to match the role. When I was preparing Jake Gyllenhaal for *Prince of Persia*, for instance, I had him training in the sand tracks in Hyde Park in London, as the script indicated that he was going to be running in the Sahara. The costume department had told me that Jake would be wearing a heavy costume during filming, so I got him to work out in a weighted vest. It's all about mimicking the conditions for the shoot environment, ensuring that the actor has the best possible preparation and is in optimum shape.

You can apply a similar thought process to your own life and fitness goals. Consider how your programme is relevant to you and your life, and how it might improve and complement your fitness. Make sure you can implement whatever you are doing into your life. If, for instance, you have young children and spend all day carrying them around, you don't want your programme to over-fatigue your muscles. It would be more beneficial to focus on stretching and recovering as you're already getting a workout from carrying your kids. Your programme should be making your life easier, not harder.

SETTING MICRO GOALS

While there is often a spontaneity to Bond on screen, the preparation for *No Time to Die* got underway over a year before shooting began, when Daniel and I first started talking about the character and the direction that the director wanted to go in. By breaking down the script, and then having discussions with Daniel, I was able to plan the training to ensure he was ready to shoot the opening chase sequence as well as the subsequent stunts. As with all the other film projects I have worked on, it's exciting to design a fitness programme based on the stunts, costumes and hand weapons, whether they're swords, shields or lightsabres.

By thinking about how much time Daniel would need to get in shape – the periodization – I knew where we had to be month by month and week by week, including planning the tough pre-production boot camps that I like to do. For your own design process, these small or incremental goals will help you to monitor your own progression.

Once you have set out where you want to be in, say, six months, you can then work back and break it down into weekly objectives. For instance, this could mean that you're going to work out four times this week, with each session lasting thirty minutes. And then next week you could add some more time, or increase the sets or reps (short for repetitions). It's important that you don't challenge yourself too much at the beginning, but that you have those regular modest goals and can feel the gradual progression.

PACE YOURSELF

Before starting a new programme with a client, I always ask them to have a physical screening. This involves getting everything checked over as that allows me to have a full understanding of their body, which aids the prevention of injuries. If you are at the start of your fitness journey, it's always a good idea to check in with a doctor. If you are looking to progress or step up a level, it never hurts to see a physiotherapist or physical therapist to find out if there are any niggles or underlying issues. A physio might give you information that allows you to tailor your programme and monitor certain parts of your body. Where possible, arrange a follow-up appointment for a few months later to discover if your body has responded.

If you push yourself too hard too quickly, it won't be sustainable. In the beginning, don't force it. Don't chase it. Let things happen naturally and organically. Daniel and I would build slowly towards the goals that I had set and you should do the same. As the first day of shooting for No Time to Die got closer, I would raise the intensity if I felt it was necessary. By this late stage, we would have been working at an extremely high level. Starting slowly doesn't mean you're any less ambitious about where you're trying to get to.

The first few weeks and months were tough when preparing for No Time to Die, just as they had been for the earlier films.

But Daniel and I knew we had the time and the right programme to achieve what we wanted because I had carefully mapped it out. The hardest thing is always getting started, but once you set off, building momentum and consistency can happen easily and quickly. If you pace yourself, you reduce the likelihood of injury and burnout. Don't skip levels; move from one to the next, making steady, incremental progress. Give yourself enough time to reach your main goals and you will get there in good time.

TRAIN EARLY

Some high-profile actors prefer to work out at 2.30 a.m., as they believe they are at their optimum at that time of the morning. You can get a mental boost from knowing you are putting in the work while others are still sleeping.

I trained Jake Gyllenhaal at 3.30 a.m. when he was shooting *Prince of Persia* in the Sahara Desert. This was partly due to the busy filming schedule, but also because we wanted to work out before the sun came up at 5 a.m., as the heat in the desert was exceptionally intense. But even outside of these extreme situations, it's very common in the film industry to be in the gym at 5 a.m., as you need time to train before travelling to set to start a day's work.

While I'm not going to suggest that you should be as zealous as some of my clients, I do believe that scheduling early sessions is the best way of ensuring that you have no interruptions and training becomes a priority at the start of the day. If you've got a workout planned for later in the day, and you're busy with work and your personal life, that training session is going to be the first thing you drop. If you know you have some physical activity timetabled for early in the morning, you won't have the chance to talk yourself out of it. I'm all for getting to sleep early so you can wake up in good time and get the work done.

LET NATURE RE-ENERGIZE YOU

When I was in the military, I recall being confined to the lower decks of an aircraft carrier for more than three weeks while carrying out my duties. I remember the euphoria of finally being allowed back into nature, which re-energized all my senses. I haven't taken nature for granted since.

Training sessions aren't just about boosting your muscle tissue, flexibility and cardiovascular fitness. Most importantly, you've got to be aware of your mental wellbeing. On long, indoor shoot days, actors may not see natural light all day – they'll arrive at the studio in the early hours, when it's dark, work all day and then leave in the evening when it's dark again.

If you have a choice of where you're going to work out, nature should always be your first choice. Being outside stimulates all your senses and has multiple benefits for your wellbeing, such as getting Vitamin D from sunlight, breathing in fresh air and having an abundance of natural distractions to keep you motivated. If you only ever work out in the gym, you're not giving yourself the natural diversity that would allow you to progress even further.

When you're outdoors, try also to make the most of your surroundings. You might usually listen to music when you're running or training in the open air, but why not press pause and see how you feel? If you take your headphones out of your ears, you'll be more alert and you can also savour the natural sounds around you – a bit of birdsong, people chatting while exercising in the park, perhaps. All these everyday sounds can make you feel connected with the here and now, and that can be just as motivational as the pumping bass of your favourite song.

CREATING CONVENIENCE

When I trained Claire Foy for *The Girl in the Spider's Web*, she wanted to do everything outside. Being in natural surroundings was great for her general wellbeing but, to be honest, the real reason we did it was because it was convenient for her – she could walk out of her front door and her session would start immediately.

Make your programme as straightforward as possible. Never give yourself an unrealistic schedule that you won't be able to maintain, such as driving to a gym that's forty-five minutes away, as you'll soon tire of the journey time and start to make excuses for not going. Like anything in life, convenience is key. It's far better to find a way of working out in or very close to your home. If training is an accessible activity, it will become part of your daily routine and you'll reach a point where it becomes second nature. If you're going to drive somewhere to exercise, try not to do that too often. Let's say your favourite yoga teacher works in a studio that's an hour or so from your home – save that for the weekend.

If you are going to travel to a gym, include the journey in your routine if possible – cycle or run there rather than getting in the car or taking the train or bus. When I'm in New York City, and feeling jet-lagged, I like to get up super early and run across Brooklyn Bridge, do a 5 a.m. spin class in Manhattan and then run back to my hotel.

Half the battle is finding what works for you, and what's convenient and efficient, because as soon as you do that, life is going to feel so much easier. People get so preoccupied by scheduling fitness around their day-to-day. But the key is making it a natural part of your daily routine. It should become so ingrained in your life that you don't even have to think about it.

You also don't have to spend hours and hours working out. I remember saying to Sam Worthington – while training him for *Wrath of the Titans* – that I only needed him for twenty minutes (his brief to me had been: 'Just the arms, mate, they're the only things on show'). I think Sam had been expecting me to suggest two-hour workouts, so he was pleasantly surprised. By shortening your sessions and upping the intensity, you're making your programme much more convenient. Benicio Del Toro was the epitome of efficiency. He would usually do twenty to thirty minutes of exercise, but on some mornings he would say to me: 'Let's do a short one today.' It's always better to do something than nothing at all.

I also often like to put the film's branding up in the gyms I create. If it's *Jurassic World*, I might dot a few dinosaur figures around, and for the *Aladdin* gym I had a huge stencil of the magic lamp on the wall. It might sound unnecessary, but it provides a constant reminder to the actors of why they're there and why they're working so hard. You might want to try doing something similar. While you might not be preparing for a major feature film, you can put up something motivational in your space – a few inspirational photos or a positive message. Always keep in mind what you're working towards; don't lose sight of the goals.

BE ADAPTABLE, BE PATIENT

When working with Donnie Yen, an incredible martial artist, on *Star Wars*, I had to be careful not to compromise his flexibility and dynamism, as speed and hand–eye coordination are an integral part of his approach. Everything I did was complementary to his existing, highly polished routine. I am always very conscious of not over-fatiguing actors before a big fight scene, so I also had to be aware of his schedule for the week ahead. Consequently, my programme for Donnie was flexible and we adjusted it to fit alongside shooting particular scenes.

In a similar way, you should tweak your schedule if your week changes. While you need some structure, because that gives you efficiency, you always have to be flexible. Your commitments are not likely to be the same from week to week, and your programming shouldn't be either.

Many people have such a rigid fitness programme that when

they're suddenly in a slightly different space in their life, they don't know how to adjust it, which is an all-or-nothing mentality. It's far better to be able to adapt and have different routines ready. That allows you to tailor your regimen and maintain a sustainable level of fitness. To keep moving forward, you need to ditch the excuses and always come up with solutions that allow you to work around your commitments and changing schedule.

Especially when you're first starting out on your fitness journey, you may not see the results of your hard work for some time. It's really important to just keep going and push through, and you will turn a corner and reach the point when you'll say to yourself: 'Wow, where did that come from?' That was my experience when training Chris Evans for *Captain America*. Suddenly, body fat is being burned away, muscle tissue is being revealed, flexibility is improving, and you're getting faster and stronger.

The hardest time during training is around six weeks into starting a new programme, which is when you reach a natural plateau. That's a good moment to take it back to the beginning and prove to yourself how much you have accomplished. I do this often with my clients as it's great for motivation. Drag it all the way back to day one. Do the workout that you did on the very first day. You'll find it easy. And that will give you a huge boost in motivation as you'll see how much progress you've made, and how achieving numerous micro goals results in major gains.

YOUR GOAL DOESN'T HAVE TO BE PHYSICAL

A lot of people don't exercise because they necessarily want to get stronger or look better, but they do so purely for their mental health and wellbeing. There are so many reasons for working out, and if that's your motivation, it's probably the best one there is.

One of my favourite things to do is to design and build bespoke gyms and spaces for clients. I was lucky enough to do that for Will Smith when he was shooting *Aladdin* at Longcross Studios near

London. He was clear that the gym wasn't just for him but for the whole cast and crew. His philosophy was that everyone he was surrounded by should have a healthy body, mind and outlook, as the fitter and healthier they were, the more productive they would be. Will thought that if everyone felt good from working out, that would result in a great movie.

The site really inspired the crew, as it had everything you could possibly wish for from a fitness setting. Will was big on exercise, and in addition to the gym equipment there was a basketball court, a 30-metre running track and a mini five-a-side football pitch, as well as an urban ju-jitsu fight area with concrete blocks around the mats. It was a place for escapism. Though I did wonder sometimes whether I had designed it a little bit too well, as the producers often had a hard time getting Will out of there and on to set.

2 | GET OUT OF YOUR COMFORT ZONE

Although many film stars lead privileged lives, surrounded by staff, when it comes to fitness no one else can do the hard work for you; you can't hire an assistant to do your dead lifts or pull-ups.

Getting Daniel in shape for *No Time to Die* took more than a year, but the boot camp was always the period that was the most intense, brutal and focused. He would have to be away from his family for much of it, which made things extra tough. But when working on Bond, Daniel was willing to put himself through boot camp and leave his comfort zone to get himself where he needed to be. If you want to achieve your personal fitness goals, you may have to do the same, but the incredible end result should provide the drive you need to get there.

WORK ETHIC

Benicio Del Toro was another actor who was keen to put in the work. I found him to be an amazing, funny guy with loads of personality, but there was a serious side to him, too, and when I trained him in London for *Guardians of the Galaxy* and a Star Wars movie, *The Last Jedi*, he gladly did short, intense daily workouts at 5 a.m. He loved wearing a purple-and-yellow LA Lakers tracksuit for our sessions – for that time of the morning it was pretty bright and always made me smile – and going for a coffee afterwards.

I was always learning from Benicio, who is prepared to work hard for short periods to maintain a good level of fitness. Like many actors, he's seeking longevity in the business and he found that training brought him energy and clarity. What I took from my time with Benicio was that short, sharp, intense workouts are incredibly effective.

Donald Glover is another example of an actor with a ferocious work ethic. He couldn't have been any more dedicated when preparing for *Solo: A Star Wars Story*. For all his talent, Donald's commitment to my programme was phenomenal – he was fitting in brief but intense workouts between being on set, writing and his other projects. I didn't realize at the time, but I was also helping him to prepare for his 'This is America' music video, which he recorded as Childish Gambino. At the time, he told me that he needed to look natural and fit, and as though he had been in the gym without being too built. I only realized what the training had been for many months later, when I happened to see the video on TV.

Felicity Jones was also meticulous with her training for *Rogue One: A Star Wars Story*. She was adamant that she wanted to do a lot of her own stunts for her role as Jyn Erso, with numerous complicated fight choreography scenes. Felicity needed a great deal of dynamic flexibility for that movie. She seemed to fill every minute of the day when she wasn't filming with some form of exercise that was going to progress her fitness, whether that was physical or mental. I've found that to be quite typical of many actors, who are forever seeking that extra element of performance which will help them to better represent the character they are playing. I also noticed this with Thandiwe Newton, who I trained for *Solo: A Star Wars Story*, that she would always make use of any spare time she had. If she suddenly had an hour free, she would work out.

While my job is to help actors achieve their required performance levels, if they wish to make big gains then they have to adopt a strong work ethic. There's no movie magic or smoke and mirrors when it comes to performance, and they're going to have to graft if they want to reach their optimum level of fitness. In my mind, if an actor is asked to sprint down a street or climb over a wall, they need to have the capability through strength and conditioning, and that's down to my coaching and their execution. That's a good lesson for all of us: to take responsibility for yourself and your own performance. Unfortunately, there's no quick fix; you need to be prepared to work for the goals that you have set yourself.

But, with willpower and dedication, you can achieve anything. From working closely with some of the world's biggest stars, I can tell you that what separates them from the rest is that they are hungry and driven, that they are willing to work hard and take it to the next level to get results.

We can learn a lot from actors about leaving your comfort zone. Sometimes you're going to have to put in the hard grind (though this is not always essential, as I explain later in the book). You also need to take some risks and try something new. Having some variety or diversity in your fitness programme is going to be of huge benefit and will help to give you progression.

DO SOMETHING NEW

When I change things up and tell an actor that they're going to use the rowing machine today and not the treadmill as usual, the response I normally receive is, 'But I've never rowed before.' That's exactly what I want: for them to be in an alien space and doing something completely new. I want them to be surprising and challenging their body.

One of the most important things to understand about the human body is that it likes to be lazy. It's lazy because it's smart; the body is always trying to conserve energy, creating the physiological patterns and muscle-firing sequences that will allow it to do that activity again more efficiently in the future. It only wants to use the essential muscles to perform that task or function, using the minimum effort and energy for maximum impact.

When you ask your body to do something for the first time, or for the first time in years, it puts stress on the central nervous system. Your body will inevitably recruit every single muscle group it has to complete the task, which is why initially it will often feel exhausting. Your brain is busy trying to figure things out, but throwing your body these curve balls is going to help give you the adaptation, or change, you need to get fit. As the brain and body work together, they work out sequences and patterns very quickly, so the next time you ask your body to perform the same task, it will recognize and understand it, and make it more efficient. You won't feel so fatigued and that is basic adaptation.

That's why I encourage people to take themselves off and try new activities and sports. It could be anything from rock climbing to yoga or boxing – you may have the fitness for your favourite activity, but as soon as you add something new your body is probably going to end up hurting. You're using patterns and recruiting muscles that you didn't realize you had.

When I trained Laura Dern for *Jurassic World*, I saw how much she embraced new information and exercises. Wanting to maintain her health and fitness throughout the production, with high levels of energy and performance, she was always looking for diversity and to learn. I provided Laura with the natural variety that would help her prepare for particular scenes.

Throwing a curve ball ultimately provides mental stimulation and relieves boredom. While some people might want to do the same thing the whole time, I prefer variety in my sessions as I've seen what a massive difference it can make.

When Daniel Craig was shooting scenes in Jamaica for *No Time to Die*, a small group of us had the chance to stay at the GoldenEye Hotel, which was Ian Fleming's old villa overlooking the sea. It's one of the most amazing places on Earth, and while

I was there I went to the beach where Ursula Andress and Sean Connery filmed that iconic scene from *Dr No*, the first Bond film from 1962. I couldn't help but feel very fortunate to be involved in the making of the Bond movies.

But another memory of that Jamaica job was getting up early to go paddleboarding or swimming with Daniel before work, which contributed to the feel-good factor of the training programme. There was very much a holiday vibe to those mornings in Jamaica, as we embraced nature while being outside and having some diversity in the sessions. Getting out of the studio and being on the road on location allows everybody to build a sense of community and camaraderie, and makes you feel as though you are part of something special. It was one of those trips that reminded me why I love my job.

It's really important that you take any opportunity to mix it up, as variety stops your fitness from being very one-dimensional. When you're not doing something completely new, you can also introduce some changes within the same exercise. Put a fresh spin on it. You can modify different aspects of an exercise and experiment with the details – for example, the number of reps you do, and the speed and tempo at which you do them. Variation engages more stabilizer muscles around the main muscles, which helps with fitness progression.

Refreshing your approach to working out also helps to stop the onset of boredom. If you can avoid feeling repetitive, you're much more likely to stay motivated and continue with your programme. And when you leave your comfort zone to try something for the first time, even if it's just a new variation on an exercise, that's going to help keep you engaged and challenged.

DON'T ALWAYS DO WHAT YOU LOVE

We all have to do things that we don't enjoy. That's certainly true of actors. Daniel doesn't love running but, unfortunately for him,

Bond is always running and it can't be avoided. At the beginning of every Bond movie, 007 is either pursuing someone or he's being chased himself, whether sprinting up and down flights of stairs, through the streets and across rooftops, or bursting through windows and smashing down doors. Daniel had to be capable of doing that time and time again, take after take. Running and changing direction was always an important element of our programme, even if it wasn't our favourite activity.

You probably don't have to work on the things you love because you're good at them already. That's the reason why you like them so much. But you should work on the things that are new to you and that are more challenging. In time, you might even find that you start to embrace an activity that you previously didn't enjoy. Sprinkle some of what you don't love into your fitness programme, as well as some of what you do. That's how you keep yourself stimulated.

You'll be surprised by what you're capable of. Don't underestimate yourself. That's a big lesson. We're all able to achieve a lot more than we think. But first we have to leave our comfort zone to realize that, as otherwise we'll never find out what's possible.

3 | TRAIN LIKE A CHILD: HAVE MORE FUN

Daniel Craig and I would start most workouts by throwing a rugby ball around for half an hour. We love a bit of rugby. Sometimes we played with a baseball. Occasionally, we kicked a football about. All good fun and it felt very natural.

Some mornings we went for a bike ride, and on others we created our own mini triathlon by adding a swim and a run. We were always conscious of having more fun when we worked out. I wanted Daniel to go back to the euphoria of childhood, the joy and the freedom you used to feel in your youth. Up to the age of about thirteen, we take our physicality for granted. As a child, you're completely uninhibited. You're climbing trees, jumping around and moving without thinking. I like actors to get back into that headspace as really that's what's required when shooting films; you want to unconsciously move and react.

Six weeks after starting a new programme, it's extremely important to inject more fun and challenges into your sessions. That's because that's the time when most people are likely to lose motivation and give up – the infamous six-week plateau. You had a burst of enthusiasm at the beginning and you're making progress, but then you get to the point where you're no longer making big gains and you start to wonder if it's all really worth it.

Maybe it's time to change things up in the form of reps, tempo and activity. The reality is that your body isn't plateauing, but transitioning and adapting. If you're going to avoid becoming a statistic, one of the many who give up after six weeks, you need to push through by having more fun.

EMBRACE YOUR INNER CHILD

Ride your bike like you're being chased. Kick a football around. Go for a swim. Play cricket. Embark on a hike. Sprint when you can – and I mean really sprint rather than go for a fast jog. Feel your body moving, your heart pumping, your blood coursing through your veins; you're feeling truly alive, maybe for the first time in a while.

I talk to a lot of my clients about being a bit childish when it comes to getting fit. It's healthy as an adult to do things that you haven't done since your younger days, as so rarely do we allow ourselves that sense of pure enjoyment. You should have that fun. It's great for your mind to go back to a time when it wasn't so clogged up with structure and responsibilities, and all-consuming stresses.

As adults, we don't use our internal feelings much to stimulate us. We use external stimulants – caffeine, alcohol and sugar – to feel euphoric and chase energy instead. But it's not too hard to remember those feelings you had as a child, when you had so much natural energy and your mental wellbeing was amazing. Training like a child is about trying to recapture the time when you had no stresses and you felt free. You'll most likely be outdoors, too, which will further enhance the experience. You'll be working hard but you'll be less conscious of it because you'll be enjoying yourself, and that helps to reduce the mental fatigue that often comes with exercise.

If you're new to working out and you start with rigid, structured sessions, that can be difficult to maintain. Staying physically and mentally flexible gives you the opportunity to adjust your sessions to suit your mood that day. That's because as a child you do everything more spontaneously, and you only do as much as you want until it's no longer fun. As well as boosting your wellbeing, training like a child allows you do to things more naturally and unconsciously in the beginning, and as you progress you will be able to easily transition into more organized workouts.

Every session doesn't have to be a grind. If you're going to achieve your fitness goals, you need to have a bit of structure around you, but some days you have to judge what type of session you feel like doing, and how intense and specific that may be. It might be more beneficial to kick a football around for half an hour. You can use training like a child as a good default for when you don't feel like a full-on session. Allow yourself the flexibility of occasionally ignoring the structured workout and being a little more free.

TRAIN WITH A FRIEND

When Daniel and I were training for the Bond movies, we decided that I was better suited to being a training buddy than a drill instructor. Every single exercise that Daniel did, I did as well (or tried to!). That made training more motivational and enjoyable for Daniel, as he wasn't going through the pain on his own. I was suffering beside him. We were taking this journey together. I think that there's a lesson there for everyone – it's always better to work out with someone as you can feed off their energy and take inspiration from them.

If you're training with a friend, you can benefit from the social side, too – humans naturally enjoy being around other humans, so spending time with someone you like is good for your general wellbeing and motivation. You can also take the chance to discuss how the session is going. And once you've made an appointment to meet – which could be once or twice a week – you feel as though you don't want to let your friend down, so you're less likely to cancel a workout.

When you're starting a new programme, it's even more beneficial to have the support of a friend or family member. You're likely to need each other more in the first few weeks, when you're adding training to your lifestyle for the first time. However, this is a two-way street as friends can certainly influence you to work out, but they can also discourage you from training.

Having a training buddy also introduces a competitive element, should you want it. You see your friend working hard alongside you and you want to do the same – or better. I've done a couple of joint sessions with Emily Blunt and her husband John Krasinski, and they become very competitive very quickly. But they also praise and motivate each other. Maybe Emily would say to John: 'Wow, I didn't realize you could do that.' And, then a few minutes later, John would say to Emily: 'How the hell are you doing that? Let me have a try.'

DO SOMETHING UNUSUAL

When you're walking or running on a treadmill, that can be repetitive as you've done it so many times before as an adult. But when was the last time that you tried to balance on one leg for as long as possible, or touch your toes, which you would have done as a child just for fun? It's fantastic for your stability, and it's also stimulating to do something for the first time in years and realize that you're capable of doing it.

I'm always conscious of making my workouts interesting and avoiding boredom. Another activity to try is a reaction game with beanbags or tennis balls. You stand with your back to a friend, and then on their call you spin around and they immediately throw the bag or ball for you to catch. These are great for hand–eye coordination and are commonly used by professional athletes who require quick reactions, such as Formula One drivers and tennis players. Never be afraid of using techniques favoured by the professionals, as anyone can try them.

4 | ACTIVATION AND DEACTIVATION

Other trainers might like to talk of a 'warm-up', but I am never really sure whether you actually warm up the muscle fibres, or whether it's more about raising your core temperature. That's why I prefer to call it 'activation', as to me it's about waking up and activating the mind and body.

It's a three-part activation. You're activating your mind to get ready to do something more intense than your usual everyday activities. You're also preparing your musculoskeletal system for work. At the same time, you're activating your cardiovascular system – raising your heart rate – to perform a task. I like to see it as making your body adopt a different attitude, switching from everyday mode into activity or athletic mode. In short, you're readying yourself for action. It's also essential, because if you don't activate your mind and change your mentality, there is an increased risk of injury as your concentration levels won't be so high.

The more often you activate, the more efficient the mind and body become at putting themselves into activity mode. Some days, you might not feel like doing a full workout, but you can still persuade yourself that you'll try the activation portion, just so you're doing something. And almost every time, you'll do that activation and your energy will kick in, allowing you to carry on and complete the full session.

I'm always looking at the methods of different athletes, examining how boxers, footballers, rugby players and other sportsmen and women activate their minds and bodies. I'm constantly absorbing new techniques and developing what I do in order to help actors get the most out of this part of the programme.

DON'T OVERLOAD

Always treat this part of your training programme as an activation and not the workout, so don't overload the muscles. Everyone's unique, and we all like to do different things to switch modes – some of us like a longer activation period, while others prefer a shorter one. But whatever you do, make sure you haven't pre-exhausted the muscles you're about to work before you get to the main training session. Some people have a tendency to go too heavy and too intense with their activation, which then doesn't allow them to maximize their workout – they need to train with their brain instead of their ego.

Normally, when actors have an action day I make them do thirty minutes of activation to prepare the body to work at a high level of intensity. But if you're about to do an intense workout, I would suggest doing around fifteen to twenty minutes of low-level activation, to make sure you are in the right mode. If you're doing a shorter or lighter workout, however, feel free to be faster and more efficient with your activation, and just spend five to ten minutes preparing.

FLICK THE SWITCH

It's vital to know how to flick the switch in your brain that says you're going from standard mode to athletic mode. In the film business, actors need to activate before shooting a stunt or action sequence as they need to make sure their mind and body are ready for what they're going to be asked to do.

Before an actor does a stunt, it is important to warm up their brain. You can't start from zero and go straight into a stunt sequence, just as an athlete wouldn't go directly on to the track and compete in their event. It's crucial that your mind and body are working in unison. Your mind needs to be as fast and as efficient as your body, otherwise you will have slower reactions and you won't look so believable on screen. We all love and feel the power of music, and when you press play and hear the start of a favourite track, that's going to release dopamine and put you on a musical high. The music is stimulating your brain and potentially increasing your focus and also raising your heart rate. Music can send a signal that it's time to work.

As an actor, an athlete or anyone who is invested in their fitness, it helps to have a clean and tidy mind. Just as a racing driver would visualize every corner of the track before getting into their car, use the same technique to imagine your workout from start to finish. If you're organized, there will be no confusion, and you will get the content and the intensity right. Ideally, you want to be able to access your emotions and turn them on and off when you need them, going from bursts of controlled, efficient aggression, with fast and dynamic movement, to calm, controlled breathing and motion.

Activating your mind can even come down to the type of stretching you do. Dynamism means more movement, and this reduces the boredom factor – so dynamic stretches are great for stimulating the mind and sending a signal that you need to switch modes. They also raise your heart rate a little because you're using your own bodyweight. Static stretching can be a bit boring and I don't feel it serves much purpose. Muscles don't like being static. They prefer to move. They need to be stimulated and for the blood to be flowing. If you're doing a static stretch, muscles aren't going to be in their natural state – they're there for actions.

In my opinion, dynamic stretches can be a useful way of getting your breathing right for when you start your workout.

Make sure you're breathing out at the time of exertion, as that helps to give you more controlled power. It also allows you to breathe more deeply and get more oxygen into the lower parts of your lungs.

Here are ten of my favourite stretches that I use over and over again with my clients:

BEAR CRAWL INTO PIGEON

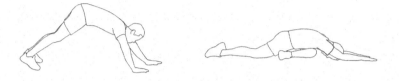

This one targets the glutes and piriformis. Stand with your feet shoulder-width apart and your hands by your sides. Gradually bend down, pivoting from the hip until your hands hit the floor in front of you. Now crawl out until you are flat in a plank position. Drive one leg forward slightly, placing your knee on the ground at a 90-degree angle and gradually moving down onto your forearms. As that stretch starts to ease, stretch your fingers out and crawl them forward so your arms are flat on the ground with your leg underneath you at 45 degrees, with your knee under your chest bone, stretching and slightly rocking from side to side. Place your hands shoulder-width apart and push yourself up, and bring your leg back to the normal starting position. Now crawl your hands back incrementally, a few inches at a time, and very slowly return to the standing position. Then place your hands on your hips and slightly rotate your hips. Take a deep breath in and out, and then repeat on the other side.

NARROW SQUAT INTO SIDE ABDUCTOR STRETCH

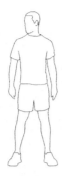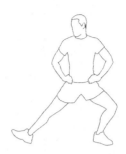

This one targets the abductor muscles. Stand with your feet shoulder-width apart. Go into squat motion and move one leg out to the side while pointing your toes in the air. Now stretch the inside of the leg, the abductor, before returning to the start position and repeating on the other side.

REVERSE LUNGE WITH HIP FLEXOR STRETCH

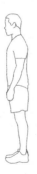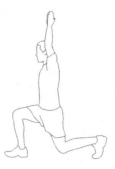

This targets the hip flexor. Stand with your feet shoulder-width apart, and then step back and lower one knee towards the ground. Your fingers are interlocked as you raise your hands above your head and lean back slightly, providing a stretch in your hip flexor. Make this more dynamic by adding a a forwards and backwards rocking motion.

ADAPTED MOUNTAIN CLIMBER WITH HAMSTRING ACTIVATION

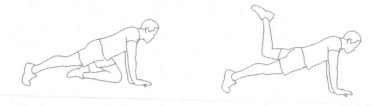

This stretch targets your glutes and hamstrings. Either use a bench or be on the floor in the push-up position. Now lift one knee and bring it up towards your elbow. Quickly bring your leg back with an adapted donkey kick, with your leg going straight up in the air bent at the knee at a 90-degree angle.

REGULAR SIT-UP WITH LUMBAR TWIST

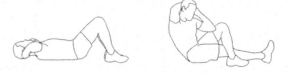

This one targets your abdominals, lower back and glutes. Lie on your back with your feet on the floor, your legs bent with raised knees and your hands on your temples. Raise yourself up and do a regular sit-up, but as you reach the end point, put both legs flat on the ground and then put one leg over the other, so that the ankle is on the outside of the knee. Put your elbow on the outside of your knee and twist until you feel a slight stretch in your lumbar in your lower back. Return to the starting position and repeat the exercise on the other side.

KNEELING TO STANDING WITH FOOT STRETCH INTO CHILD'S POSE

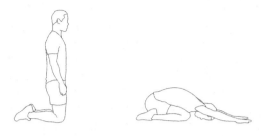

A great one for targeting the feet and toes, quads and glutes, as well as your back. Kneel on the floor, then move to a standing position. Go back down onto your knees with your feet tucked underneath and sit back on your heels, allowing the feet to stretch, and hold that for around thirty seconds. Turn the feet so they are flat on the ground, and bring your forehead to the floor, with your arms stretched out in front of you, to move into Child's Pose, a yoga position. Hold that for around twenty seconds.

QUAD STRETCH REVERSE LUNGE KNEE PULL

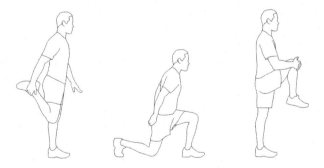

This is to stretch the quads and glutes, and is also good for balance. Stand up and raise one leg behind you in a normal quad stretch, clasping the ankle. Hold for thirty seconds and then allow that leg to go backwards into a reverse lunge, with the knee touching the floor. Return to the start position, raising your knee in front of you, clasping it with both hands and then pulling it in tight. Now do the other leg.

SIDE SPIDER CRAWL

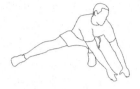

Use this one for quads, glutes and abductors. Squat down with your hands in front of you. Crawl to the side in that squatted position and then crawl back. That's it!

PEDAL TO STANDING

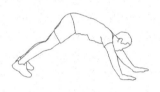 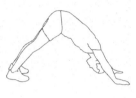 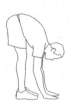

A good one for the calves. Put yourself in the pike position, so hands flat on the ground and bottom in the air. Pedal your feet – left, right, left, right – so you always have one foot in the air. Walk that pedal forward until your feet are between your hands, and then stand up nice and slowly.

PLANK TO PIKE INTO COBRA

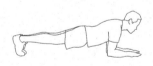 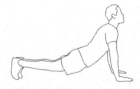

Finally, just for the abdominals. Start in the plank position, with your elbows on the floor and lying on your forearms. Raise your hips into the air. Then bring your hips down so they are an inch off the ground. Go into the cobra position where your chest comes forward, and look up slightly.

DEACTIVATION

This is the opposite of what you did with your activation – you're switching your mode back, coming out of activity mode and trying to bring the body back to its natural state. You're returning to that generic state by bringing your heart rate down and doing multidirectional drills, plus general relaxation and breathing techniques. This time also allows you to think about and prepare for what you're going to do after your workout. Nine times out of ten, this will involve hydration and nutrition, as the best time to refuel is in the twenty-to-thirty-minute window after you have finished training. You could also use this time for a little bit of meditation and to check in with yourself.

Stretching is great for mindfulness – it should help you to get into the right headspace after a workout. You're allowing your body to go into more of a rested state, with a lowered heart rate, and that helps you to reset. Stretching allows you to mark the end of a session – you're signalling to your body and mind that the physical activity is over and you're about to move on to the next part of your day. Stretching can feel good, and if something feels good, you should do it.

One breathing technique is to sit cross-legged with your elbows on your knees, as if you're in a meditational position. Feel your heart rate lower as you become more conscious of your breathing. Focus on filling the lower third of your lungs. Most of us do very shallow breathing when we exercise and we don't fill up the lungs completely. But as you deactivate, try to get as much oxygenated blood into your system as possible, which means filling every part of your lungs. Do that ten to fifteen times and you'll be in an almost Zen-like state.

Now do a ten-second sprint on the spot as that's going to reactivate everything again. You'll feel invigorated and ready for the rest of your day.

5 | MY GO-TO 5–2 METHOD

I like to think of this as the Holy Grail of fitness programming. The 5–2 is my go-to method that I use with the majority of the actors I work with, as you will see with the workouts that I've included in this book. The reason I like it is that it's given me the best results in the shortest space of time and it's adaptable – once you are familiar with it, you can take it anywhere, to any gym, home or outdoor setting.

You might be wondering why it is called the 5–2 method – very simply, it's because it involves five different exercises and two-minute bursts of cardio in between.

I tend to use a whiteboard in the gym when planning the workout, but you might prefer to write yours on a piece of paper or type it into your phone. In the left-hand column, note down your five exercises for that particular workout, and on the right side you can write down your cardio. Let's call your five exercises A, B, C, D and E. You begin with Exercise A and then do two minutes of your chosen cardio. You then add a second exercise to the first – Exercises A and B – followed by two more minutes of cardio. Then Exercises A, B and C before two minutes of cardio, after which Exercises A, B, C and D plus the two minutes of cardio, and finally Exercises A, B, C, D and E, and cardio again.

For the cardio elements, I like running and interval sprinting, boxing (hitting the pads) and explosive, powerful movements known as plyometrics (examples include skipping, hopping and lunging). If you have access to other equipment such as battle ropes – which are long, weighted ropes – that adds great variety. You can do almost anything as long as it raises your heart rate and creates intensity.

In my experience, this 5–2 method is a brilliant way of working efficiently and generating intensity as the only rest you get is when you're quickly transitioning from one exercise to another, or to the cardio.

Exercise A
Cardio
Exercise A Exercise B
Cardio
Exercise A Exercise B Exercise C
Cardio
Exercise A Exercise B Exercise C Exercise D
Cardio
Exercise A Exercise B Exercise C Exercise D Exercise E
Cardio

Whichever one you're doing, the intensity is high throughout the workout. I sometimes see people in the gym who do half an hour on the treadmill when they are training at high intensity, and then the rest of the workout is at a much lower level, with lots of rest between exercises. If you're looking for a lower intensity workout, that's fine, but with my programmes, efficiency and intensity are always key. This 5–2 method is going to help you to improve your time and energy capabilities – it gives you more bang for your buck as you're getting a sprinkling of strength alongside a measure of cardio.

There are two different kinds of muscle fibres in your body: fast twitch and slow twitch. With this method, you're targeting the fast-twitch muscle fibres – which help you with an explosive activity such as sprinting – as well as the slow-twitch fibres – for endurance, such as running a marathon. By targeting both types, you don't become so one-dimensional in your fitness. You can go for longer distances as well as for shorter bursts, which translates really well into everyday life. When using this 5–2 method, be aware that you can use as much resistance as you like, including cables and bodyweight for variety. Nothing is off the table.

BE FLEXIBLE

Don't be afraid to adjust the workout based on how you are feeling each day, or depending on your short-term and long-term goals. One option is to change the order in which you do the exercises, which makes a difference as you're going to be doing Exercise A much more than Exercises D and E. If you're looking for a workout that is more cardiovascular, use a plyometric for Exercise A. If you're feeling tired or jet-lagged, put that plyometric last as Exercise E. In time, you will learn which exercises work better for you, and also which order gives you the most benefit on any given day.

You can easily adjust the 5–2 method to suit you, which I think is why my clients have been so happy with it. It's very simple to add elements or to take them away, depending on how you're feeling and what you're trying to achieve. If you want to create a little more muscle tissue, you can remove the more dynamic exercises and instead do more high-resistance and compound exercises.

You can even play around with the numbers to help you to achieve your objectives. If your goal is more strength-based, you could increase the number of exercises to create an 8–2 workout. Or if your aim is linked to endurance – such as when you're training for a marathon – you could go up to three minutes of cardio for a 5–3 workout.

COMPOUND EXERCISES

I always try to use compound exercises as part of my workouts because they recruit more than one muscle group. You use the main muscle group and also the stabilizing muscles around that group, giving you efficient intensity as well as the potential to create lean muscle tissue (cultivating lean muscle tissue is like looking after a rare plant – you have to feed it, water it and let it grow!). These types of exercises also elevate your heart rate, which gives you a bit of a metabolic boost and adds to your calorie burn.

Compound exercises allow you to be more efficient with your time, body and mind. They are very motivational as you can easily monitor your progress and you tend to advance very quickly as you're hitting the body in so many different ways. Squats, pull-ups and bench presses are good examples. When you use your own bodyweight, that's almost always a compound exercise.

They are much more useful than isolation exercises, in which you're only working one muscle group. With compound exercises, you don't have to keep adding exercises to your workout, which becomes very time-consuming and increasingly difficult to sustain as your muscles have already been used and partially fatigued. It's this efficient approach that gives you sustainability.

6 | CREATE YOUR OWN FITNESS PROGRAMME

Through the course of this book, I'm going to be sharing with you the workouts that I designed and implemented for some of the biggest names in cinema. Many of my past workouts are still stored in my brain – I have a library in my head of the exercises I used with each actor. If you mention a film I worked on, even one that was released more than ten years ago, I think about the movement, the performance and the aesthetics, and then I'll recall how I trained that person. I hope you will be inspired by these workouts, and that today you'll start the process of moving, feeling and looking like an athletic movie star.

One of the most important takeaways from this book is that you should create a programme that really works for you. While you might find that one of these workouts inspires you and feels just right, it might also be the case that you find yourself using more than one, depending on your progression and what you feel like doing on any given day. Why not draw inspiration from Blake Lively on Monday, from Léa Seydoux on Wednesday and from Bryce Dallas Howard on Friday? Or, in the same week, you could exercise and be inspired by Daniel Craig, Chris Evans and John Boyega.

And don't think you have to stick to exactly how I trained these actors; let these workouts inspire you, but feel free to make these your own and put your own twist on them. You could also combine elements of two or more workouts. I'm providing you with a toolbox: you should always create your own fitness programme because that will give you the best chance of achieving your personal goals.

You'll see that almost all of the workouts have five exercises, as I used my go-to 5–2 method. My method is flexible and you can play around with the numbers to discover what suits you best.

Whatever your fitness level, I hope that you'll find lots of useful guidance in these various workouts. Whether you're a beginner or at a more advanced stage, you can modify an exercise to suit your current capabilities. These sessions are typical of what I did with these clients to prepare them for particular movies, but of course I often changed things up and added in new elements to the routines, and you can do this, too. Also included in these sections are the activations (commonly known as warm-ups) I did with actors before we got into the workouts themselves, especially before athletic scenes, to wake up and prepare their bodies and minds for the training to come.

DANIEL CRAIG FOR
NO TIME TO DIE

H

Daniel and I always found it motivational to work out with each other. We have always seen each other as **TRAINING PARTNERS** rather than trainer and client. That's just what works for us. I would design the workout and then we would implement it together. You can, of course, always exercise on your own, but if you've got the opportunity to train with someone else, you should take it.

When you're working out with someone else, don't just stand around watching them train – always be doing something yourself. **USE YOUR TIME**. I don't believe in rest phases during a workout.

Take some time to plan and prepare before starting this workout. I find it helpful to have all your kit laid out and ready to go so you can **BE EFFICIENT WITH YOUR TIME** and not lose any intensity while training.

Even when you're starting out on your fitness journey, you can still train like James Bond. This workout is typical of the programmes I created for Daniel Craig to condition him for *No Time to Die*. I devised this upper-body workout – which prioritizes the push-pull movements with the chest and back, as well as the abdominals, arms and obliques – to prepare Daniel for the stunt room and for the sequences in the film itself. Because of its intensity, it also helped him to achieve the high level of fitness he needed to get through a brutal filming schedule, with long days and nights on set. By the time the main shoot began, Daniel was the fittest he had ever been – and he was in his early fifties. We continued to use this workout during filming to maintain that level of fitness.

Now it's your turn: this sequence of exercises will maximize your results, boosting your own strength and endurance. It's a dynamic workout, encompassing all elements of fitness, and targets important muscle groups in the upper body. While the other workouts I have shared in this book follow my go-to 5–2 method, this one is a little different; it's a superset approach that allowed me to train with Daniel, which is what he wanted.

If you're at a basic level of fitness, you can do this *No Time to Die* workout within your limits and capabilities. Feel free to make adjustments – just change the weights and the reps and the sets accordingly. Like all the other training programmes I have developed, you can tweak as you see fit, depending on how much time you have and how you're feeling on a particular day.

Daniel and I would do this upper-body workout twice a week. This was part of a programme that also included a twice-weekly session with more cardio and movement-based content, as well as a pure legs and cardio workout. I recommend that you also incorporate other activities into your plan. That could be yoga, swimming, a bike ride or any ball sport. Anything you enjoy that raises your heart rate. Daniel loved being outside whenever possible, which is a great distraction and also fantastic for your wellbeing.

ACTIVATION AND CARDIO

Daniel and I would start by throwing a rugby ball or baseball around. We did that because it was fun and also because that allowed me to have a conversation with Daniel to assess how he was feeling that day and what his expectations were. I would ask him whether he had slept well, if he had any niggles or concerns, and whether there was anything he didn't want to do during the workout. That feedback would determine what we did – depending on how Daniel was feeling, we could add or take away certain elements. Activation might also include getting on the bike for ten minutes – it's all about preparing to work.

NO TIME TO DIE UPPER-BODY WORKOUT

Each of the five supersets is made up of an Exercise A and an Exercise B. If you're training with a friend, you each do one of the exercises in the same superset, and then immediately swap over. Daniel and I would typically use a rep range of 15 to 25 for each exercise, but if you're just starting out please adjust to your capability. Daniel and I would also try to stretch and hydrate between each superset.

SUPERSET 1
A: LOW TO HIGH CABLE CHEST FLY

This is one of my favourite ways to start any chest workout as it utilizes multiple muscle groups. You're using lots of stabilizing muscles, including abdominals and lower back, and there's also good arm movement. For this exercise you will need a typical cable machine that you would find in most gyms.

- Stand in the middle of the cables with your back to them. Hold one cable in each hand with your arms out straight and take two steps forward so you're in the split-squat stance (one leg in front of the other).
- Bring the cables up with soft elbows so they reach your forehead.
- Contract the chest muscle for around two seconds and return to the start position.

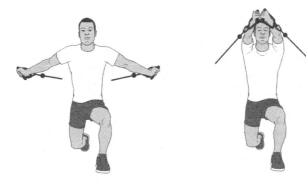

B: ABDOMINAL ROLLOUT

This is another favourite of mine. I like it because you're using almost every element of your core – abdominals, obliques and lower back – both isometrically (when a muscle is under constant tension) and concentrically (hold, squeeze and release). For this, you need an ab roller or a barbell on the floor with weight plates at both ends.

- Start off in a kneeling position with the roller in front of you, and hold it with both hands. Cross your ankles for stability.
- Roll yourself out into a stance in which you're engaging your core, hold for two seconds and return to the start position.
- As you progress, you'll be able to go further and hold for longer until you can almost get completely horizontal.
- Utilize different angles and body postures for constant variety.

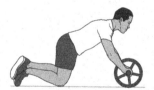 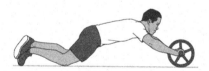

SUPERSET 2
A: BOSU MOUNTAIN CLIMBER PUSH-UP

This is one of my go-to exercises as it uses multiple elements of the body: strength from the push-up; core as it's unstable; and dynamic movement from the knee drive. All of this creates the perfect dynamic exercise which will enhance your stability.

- Go into the push-up position, clasping each side of the BOSU ball, with your feet shoulder-width apart. You need to be horizontal, engaging your core and glutes.
- Bring each knee in towards your chest and then return to the start position.
- Lower yourself down until your chest touches the BOSU for a count of three seconds and then return to the start position for three seconds.

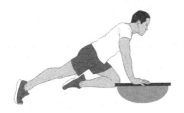
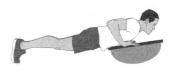

B: TRADITIONAL PULL-UP

Bodyweight exercises are probably the most difficult to master and the hardest for trainers to teach, but they are the best barometer of upper-body strength gains.

- Using an overhand grip, put your hands on the pull-up bar and position them just over shoulder-width apart.
- Cross your ankles and raise your heels until they are at a 90-degree angle – this will stop you from rocking around and ensure you engage the right muscles.
- Pull yourself up until your chin is slightly above the bar. Return to the start position.

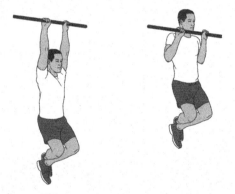

If you struggle with this exercise, you could put a bench or a chair beneath the pull-up bar, which will enable you to jump up before you slowly let yourself down.

SUPERSET 3
A: RUSSIAN TWIST

Adding an exercise with a rotation and twist is a great way of mixing things up. With the Russian twist, you will be moving more laterally. You'll get some resistance and rotation, and you'll be working the lower part of your abdominals. Lots of things will be happening all at once.

- Sit on a mat holding a resistance item – this could be a medicine ball, kettlebell, dumbbell or plate – with your legs in front of you at a 45-degree angle and your ankles crossed.
- Lift your legs 6 inches off the ground. Twist to the left, moving the resistance item so it touches the floor, and then return to the start position.
- Twist to the right and lower the item until it touches the floor on that side.

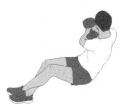
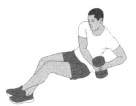

B: SIDE OBLIQUES BEND

Obliques, which are located on the sides of your abdominal muscles, are quite an overlooked muscle group but should be trained like any other. When developed correctly, they can be aesthetically pleasing when your body fat starts to drop.

- Choose your resistance item – it could be a kettlebell, plate or dumbbell. Stand with your legs shoulder-width apart and hold the weight in one hand with a straight arm, and place the other hand on top of your head.
- Allow your body to lean to the side with the resistance until you feel as though your core, abdominals and obliques are engaged, and your resistance item is below knee level.
- Return to the starting position. Try lifting heavier weights as your fitness increases. You can introduce some variation by swapping the resistance item for a band or cable above your head.

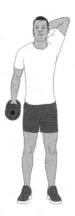 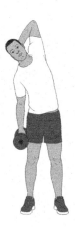

SUPERSET 4
A: TRX ROW AND CURL

The TRX is a great bit of kit to travel with and adds diversity to your workout. It's basically a strap that you can hang from a door or ceiling with loops for hands or feet at either end. I like to use this in a matrix form, doing one back row and then moving straight into a bodyweight bicep curl. You're creating intensity and fatigue through two muscle groups.

- Stand in front of the TRX with your arms locked out and your hands in a pistol grip. Walk backwards until you find the right gradient of resistance and bodyweight that you need.
- Do a rowing motion, pulling towards you with your elbows tucked by your sides so your shoulder blades are retracted, and then return to the start position.
- For the bicep curl, turn your hands so that your palms are facing up and then bring your arms to your forehead.
- Return to the original position and back to the pistol grip.
- As you progress, you can adjust the angle that you're leaning back at until you're almost horizontal.

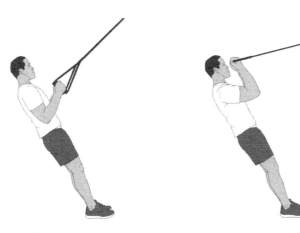

B: BODYWEIGHT DIPS

Like the traditional pull-up, this workout technique is a great barometer of strength. There is no better feeling than being able to dip your own bodyweight repetitively.

- Jump onto the dip bars with your elbows locked behind you, your ankles crossed, your legs at 90 degrees and your chest high.
- Focus in front of you as you lower your body down until your elbows are at 90 degrees.
- Return to the original position.
- You can add resistance by holding a dumbbell or a plate between your legs.

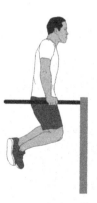 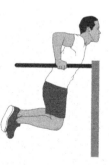

SUPERSET 5
A: HANGING LEG RAISE AND WINDSCREEN WIPER

This exercise is a great variation and complements the previous core exercises. The windscreen wiper element incorporates isometric core through abdominals, obliques and intercostals (the muscles between your ribs), giving you great detail around those muscle groups.

- Hang off the pull-up bar using an overhand grip. Lock out your arms and gradually take your feet off the ground.
- Bring your knees up to your chest and then return to the start position.
- Increase the intensity of this exercise by lightly touching the floor with your feet.
- For the windscreen wiper, with your knees to your chest, rotate your knees 45 degrees to the left, turning back to the start position and then rotating them 45 degrees to the right, and then returning to the start position. This can be adapted to your ability: add resistance by holding a dumbbell between your feet or by simply keeping your legs straight.

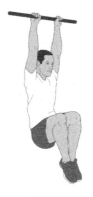 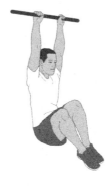

B: REVERSE BOSU CABLE RETRACTION

The BOSU ball helps you to improve your stability while you use the cables for resistance, which leads to great postural development. It's one of my go-to exercises for actors who need to film complex, choreographed stunt sequences.

- Stand on the BOSU, hard side up, facing the cable machine.
- With the cables set in a mid-position, cross your right hand over your body and grab the cable on the left-hand side. Now your left hand goes over and grabs the right-hand cable. Your arms are crossed.
- Maintain soft knees and find a focal point on the wall.
- Move your arms back into a crucifix position, squeezing and then retracting the shoulder blades while maintaining stability. Count to four and return to the original position.

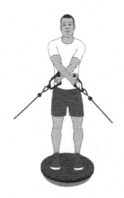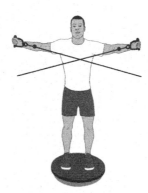

DANIEL'S WORKOUT

SUPERSET 1

Exercise A: Low to high cable chest fly x 25

Exercise B: Abdominal rollout x 25

Stretch/hydrate

SUPERSET 2

Exercise A: BOSU mountain climber push-up x 25

Exercise B: Traditional pull-up x 25

Stretch/hydrate

SUPERSET 3

Exercise A: Russian twist x 25

Exercise B: Side obliques bend x 25 on each side

Stretch/hydrate

SUPERSET 4

Exercise A: TRX row and curl x 25

Exercise B: Bodyweight dips x 25

Stretch/hydrate

SUPERSET 5

Exercise A: Hanging leg raise and windscreen wiper x 25

Exercise B: Reverse BOSU cable retraction x 25

Stretch/hydrate

LÉA SEYDOUX FOR
NO TIME TO DIE

H

I imagine Léa's workout will appeal to a lot of women reading this book. This simple workout will improve your **STRENGTH, STAMINA AND POSTURE** – it's a great all-rounder, and that's exactly what Léa needed for *No Time to Die*.

Léa never liked to do long workouts – she preferred short, **INTENSE SESSIONS**. If you're also pushed for time, this workout is quick and efficient, and if you're as **DEDICATED** as Léa was, you'll see the results very quickly.

Over the past twenty years, I've worked with a few Bond girls, going all the way back to Denise Richards in *The World is Not Enough* and Halle Berry and Rosamund Pike in *Die Another Day*. Bond girls sometimes have to do something quite specific for the role – when Rosamund played Miranda Frost she had to be able to fence, so I conditioned the right muscle groups to enable her to do that. But one thing is always at the forefront of my mind when I'm training female actors for these Bond films: to never be too extreme with their workouts. It's about great posture, elegance and movement. That was my philosophy when preparing Léa Seydoux for her role as Doctor Madeleine Swann in *No Time to Die*, the second film we worked on together after *Spectre*.

Léa's character wasn't meant to look overly athletic. I had to be sure she was physically capable of playing the part, as there was a lot of running and stunts throughout a long and demanding shoot, but I didn't want her to have too much muscle tissue. Maintaining her health and energy was the priority. Like all Bond girls, Léa needed to project great confidence on screen, and hopefully some of this would come from her fitness programme.

While I spent more than a year training Daniel Craig for *No Time to Die*, I had much less time with Léa because her role was less physical than Daniel's. The goal for Léa, which we ultimately achieved, was for her to be fast, efficient and full of energy. Now you too can train like a Bond girl.

ACTIVATION AND CARDIO

To wake up her body and mind, I liked Léa to start with some boxing on the pads, sprinting, box jumps and sidesteps. She would also do some walking lunges before going back to pad work and a sprinkling of BOSU push-ups. This type of activation allows you to go from strength to cardio to stretching, which meant Léa was activating every muscle group and getting everything moving. Before an athletic scene, I would get her to hit the pads, which would introduce some aggression and enhance her hand–eye coordination, while some skipping would give her cardio and coordination.

From sprinting on the treadmill and burpees to the SkiErg machine (like a stand-up rowing machine) and the bike, I asked Léa to do as many different types of cardio as possible. That stimulated different parts of her body and her brain, so she didn't get bored.

Burpees are a great explosive exercise for any actor in an action movie. You're going to get knocked to the floor, and so you need to be able to respond and recover quickly. If you're too slow at getting back to your feet, you're not going to look athletic or capable. Ideally, you want to be able to spring straight back up and move across the ground quickly. There was also lots of sprinting because there is a great deal of running in these films.

LÉA'S 5–2 WORKOUT

BOSU SQUATS

A regular squat without a BOSU ball is a great exercise in itself; when you do it on top of the hard side of a BOSU, it adds an extra instability dimension. You're recruiting lots of different muscle groups and working your stability.

- Stand on a BOSU with your feet just over shoulder-width apart, with your toes pointing slightly outwards.
- Lower yourself until your knees are at a 90-degree angle and hold for a count of four.
- Explode back through your heels to return to the start position.

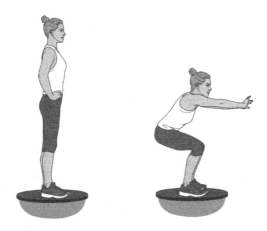

BOSU LUNGES

With these lunges, you're working the power muscles that are going to help your sprinting. You're also training your legs independently – one and then the other – which helps to avoid imbalances in your body.

- With the BOSU hard side up, put one foot in the middle while keeping the other leg parallel behind you. Your fingers should be touching either side of the BOSU as if you are in a sprinting position, parallel with the foot.
- Bring the rear leg forward so you're standing, and then raise the knee of the same leg to 90 degrees so you're standing on one leg.
- Return to the start position, in which your leg is directly behind you and your fingers return to touching the BOSU.
- Change to the other leg and repeat.

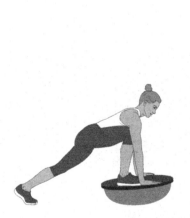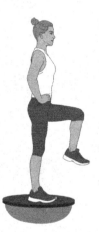

BOSU STEPOVERS

These stepovers are great for working the glutes and quads, and for building up speed and agility. The first two exercises were linear, so now it's time for a lateral one, as the body needs to move in different planes – from side to side as well as forwards and backwards.

- Place the BOSU soft side up. Stand to the side of it and put one foot in the middle.
- Skip over to the other side, replacing the foot on the BOSU with the other.
- As the foot lands on the other side, go into a slight squat.
- Skip back to the other side.
- Do this rhythmically with your hands clenched in front of you and your chest high.

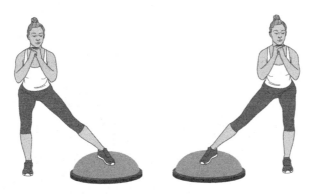

BOSU CLOCK

Léa had to be able to move quickly. This exercise helped her with swiftness of movement, and you'll find that it's also great for your own spatial awareness and ability to engage multiple muscle groups.

- With the BOSU hard side up, stand on it on your right leg with the other one in the air, around 6 inches off the ground – start with that foot pointing out in front of you.
- Move around the clock with the foot that's in the air, going from 12 o'clock to 3 o'clock to 6 o'clock to 9 o'clock. Use the heel as the 'marker' for 12 o'clock and 3 o'clock, and the toe for 6 o'clock, while for 9 o'clock your leg goes behind the other one.
- Change to your left leg and repeat.

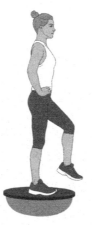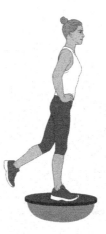

BOSU CATCHES

This exercise is great for improving your coordination, speed and agility.

- Stand on one leg on a BOSU ball with the hard side up. If this is new to you, place both feet shoulder-width apart on the BOSU.
- Engage your glutes and abdominals, and keep your knees soft or bent. Put your hands out in front of you and look up.
- A training partner throws the tennis ball, Pilates ball or weighted beanbag at you in various positions: high to low and from left to right.
- After catching and throwing the ball back, return to the original position, ready for the next throw.

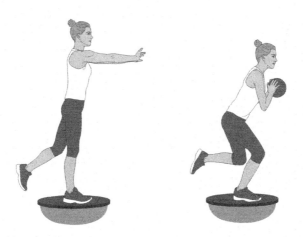

LÉA'S WORKOUT

BOSU squats x 25 reps

Cardio

BOSU squats x 20 reps

BOSU lunges x 20 reps on each side

Cardio

BOSU squats x 15 reps

BOSU lunges x 15 reps on each side

BOSU stepovers x 15 reps on each side

Cardio

BOSU squats x 10 reps

BOSU lunges x 10 reps on each side

BOSU stepovers x 10 reps on each side

BOSU clock x 10 reps

Cardio

BOSU squats x 8 reps

BOSU lunges x 8 reps on each side

BOSU stepovers x 8 reps on each side

BOSU clock x 8 reps

BOSU catches x 8 reps

Cardio

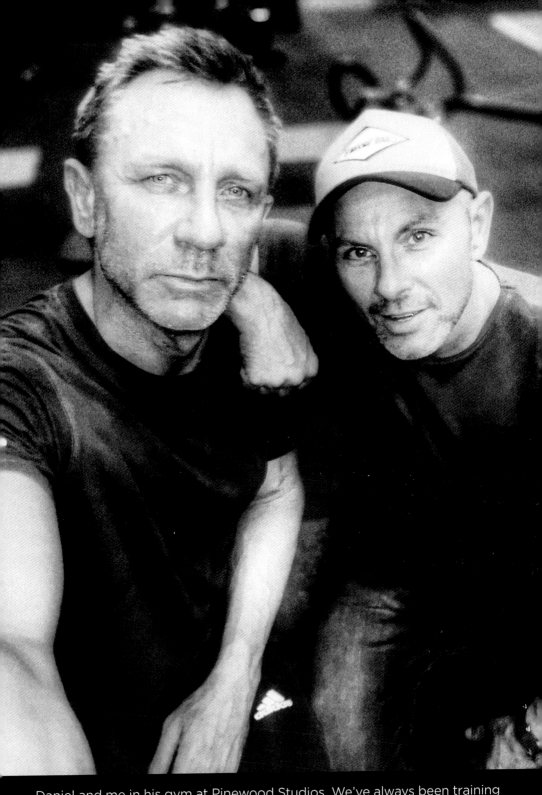

Daniel and me in his gym at Pinewood Studios. We've always been training partners – I did every rep he did when he was preparing for *No Time to Die*

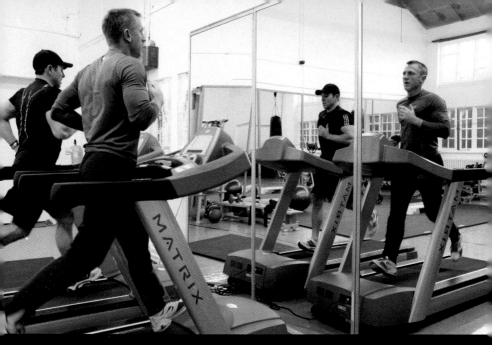

ABOVE. Being Bond means doing lots of running – Daniel needed to build a cardio base in his gym at Pinewood. This photo was taken during training for *Skyfall*.

BELOW. The English weather meant that Daniel and I often had to do his sprint drills inside his gym rather than outside on a track.

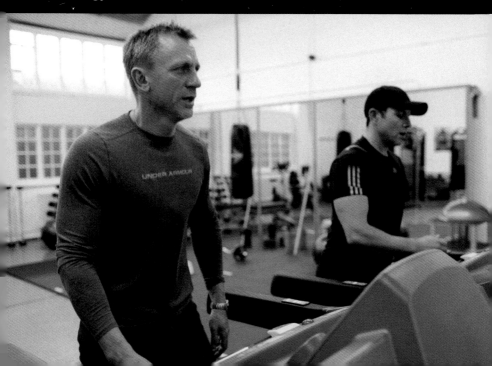

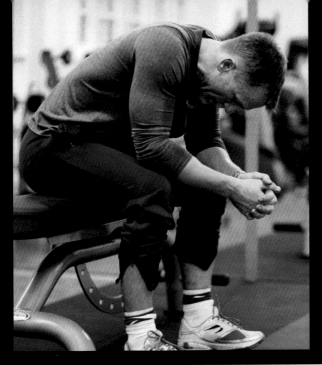

LEFT. Resting and recovering are key to improving your athletic ability.

BELOW. One of the rewards for all the hard graft was this iconic shot of Daniel emerging from the water in *Casino Royale*.

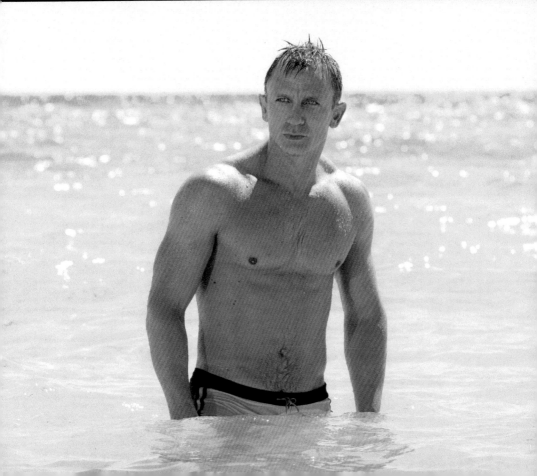

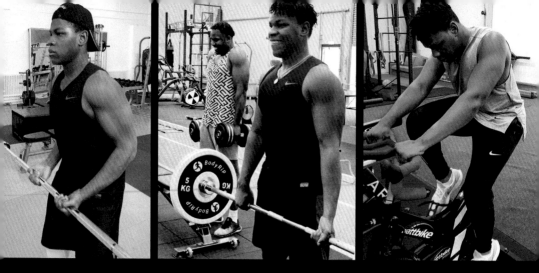

ABOVE. Preparing John Boyega for *Star Wars* – he had to move as though he had been trained as a stormtrooper.

BELOW. John on the run with Daisy Ridley in a scene from *Star Wars: Episode VII – The Force Awakens*, putting all that training to good use.

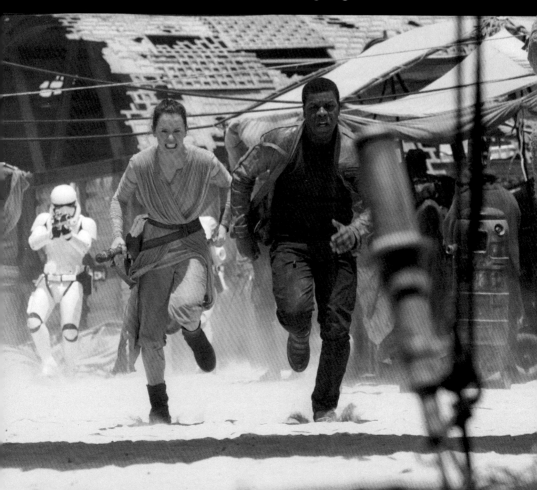

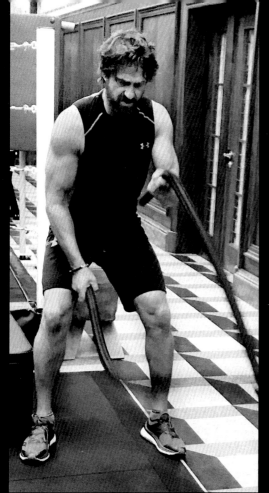

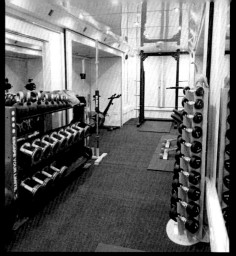

LEFT. Gerard Butler putting in the work as he prepared for *Angel has Fallen*.

ABOVE RIGHT. The workout trailer I designed for Chris Pratt for *Jurassic World*.

BELOW. On the press tour for *No Time to Die*, shooting a video with YouTuber Hailey Sani in Los Angeles.

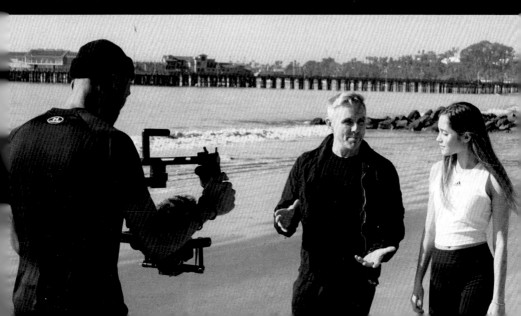

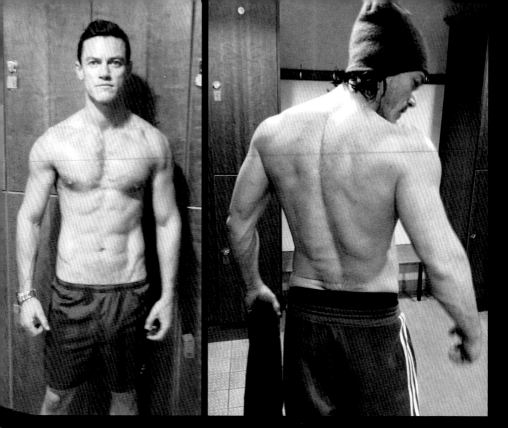

ABOVE AND RIGHT. Luke Evans' transformation for *Dracula*. His back had to look as though he was capable of flying – his character had his wings snapped off his back.

BELOW. Will Smith asked me to design and build his gym for *Aladdin*, which included a huge stencil of a magic lamp on the wall for motivation.

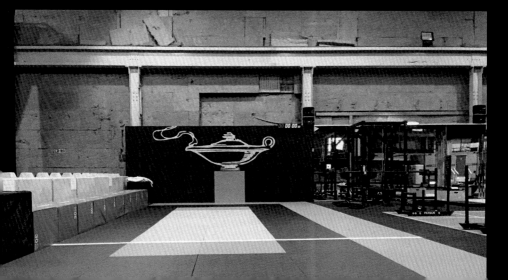

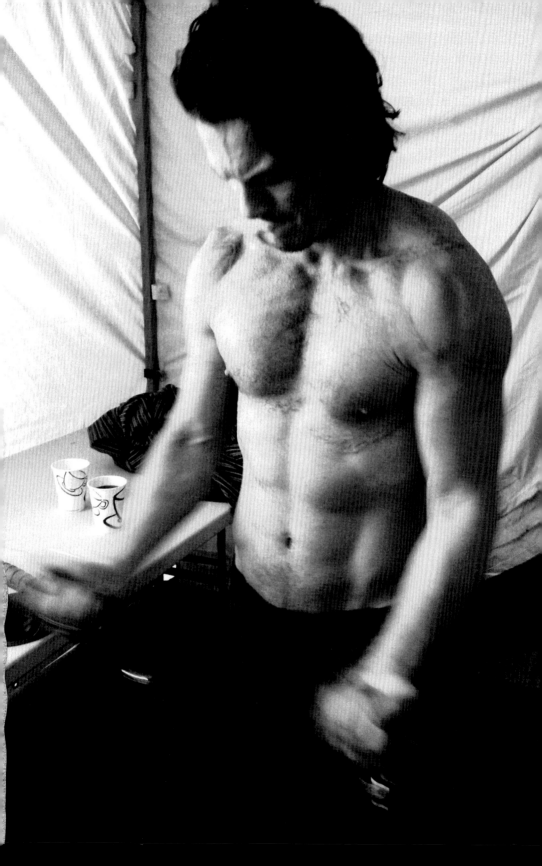

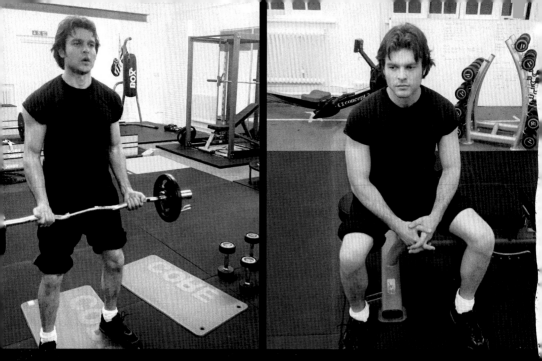

ABOVE. Alden Ehrenreich getting ready to play Han Solo in *Solo: A Star Wars Story* – he was trying to emulate Harrison Ford's physicality and demeanour in the original films, which was no small task.

BELOW. Alden looking the part during the filming of *Solo*.

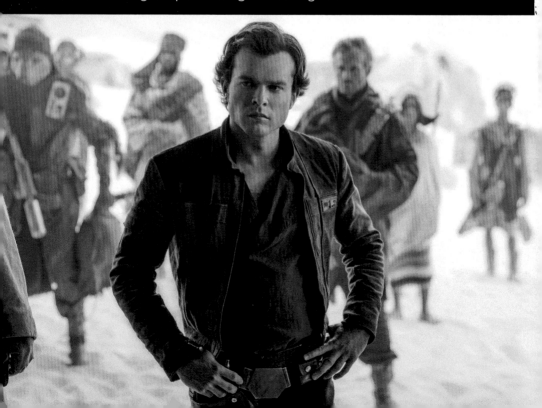

CHRIS EVANS FOR *CAPTAIN AMERICA*

H

The most inspirational thing about Chris wasn't his physical transformation; it was his **MENTALITY**. He showed what's possible when you're dedicated, and you get up and do the work.

Chris understood why you ideally want to have a **BALANCED PHYSIQUE**. When he came to me, he was slightly imbalanced from the workouts he did during his college days, which is really common – the focus had been on the chest, biceps and abs for years. While you can train those vanity muscles, you shouldn't forget to **WORK ON THE MUSCLES THAT YOU CAN'T SEE**, especially your back.

Turning a human into a Marvel superhero, a character that had previously only existed on the pages of a comic book, is about as challenging a transformation as you're going to get in the movie business.

It's very easy to draw muscles on a page. You can make them as big and as defined as you like, and you can also draw a skinny waist while you're at it. That's the Marvel Cinematic Universe, where you're only limited by your imagination; it's very different in the real world, when you're actually having to build and sculpt that muscle tissue.

On the first *Captain America*, I was lucky to speak with Stan Lee, one of the creators of Marvel, who gave me his vision. I also spoke to director Joe Johnston, who laid out all his visual references for how he imagined Chris should move and look as Captain America.

It wasn't just storyboards that Joe showed me. At one meeting, he even brought models into the room with him so he could demonstrate to me what he liked about their bodies and what I should be aiming for with Chris. Joe told me what kind of six-pack he needed with Chris, and how the obliques should look, and what type of chest he was hoping for. Joe wanted to ensure that I got the proportions right with Chris. You can see from the comic-book character that Captain America is very muscular and capable with big arms, wide chest and a six-pack. That was what we needed to emulate. There was also lots of focus on the back, as Joe wanted Chris to look as though he was permanently carrying a shield – almost as if the shield was part of his back.

The transformation took a year. To make the process a little easier, I stayed just two blocks from Chris in Boston – that meant I could quickly cycle over to his place or meet him at the gym. I tried to do as much as possible in the first six or seven months, with two sessions a day. It was gruelling, but I was able to let him get on with his life, and he was also shooting a different movie at the same time. When Chris was finding it really tough, I would tell him to hang in there and be patient.

The programme gave Chris the depth and tone of muscle that he needed. From an aesthetic standpoint, I prefer it when a muscle has a lot of depth, and you can see when it moves and contracts naturally rather than looking bloated and watery, as movement and lines are always captured on camera. The pod scene in particular was very aesthetic, with Chris emerging from the pod as Captain America, having gone in as Skinny Steve Rogers. To play Captain America, Chris needed speed and agility. He had to be highly dynamic, with super-quick reactions and amazing hand–eye coordination as well. You can't just build someone to look like that; you need to build someone to perform like that. The aesthetic was key for that film, but it always comes back to performance.

I'll never forget the day they shot that pod scene. It was a big day for Chris but also an important day for me. I was standing on set next to Stan Lee, with both of us looking at Chris, and Stan's words to me were: 'Now that's Captain America.'

ACTIVATION AND CARDIO

Chris would often jump on the treadmill to walk on an incline for ten or fifteen minutes, or he would get on the bike. He also did lighter sets of the exercises that we were going to do later. I'm always conscious that I'm taking up a fair amount of time from people who are extremely busy, which is why I try to allow an actor to multitask. If I was asking Chris to do forty-five to sixty minutes of cardio, I would make sure that sometimes he could be sitting on a bike in the gym with his laptop open in front of him to allow him to read his script simultaneously. Sometimes, however, I need clients to do some more high-intensity cardio, and so during those times multitasking isn't really possible.

CHRIS'S 5–2 WORKOUT

DEAD LIFT

This was the exercise that Chris found the toughest, but it was also the one which was most important for his transformation. A heavy dead lift stimulates a lot of the central nervous system, which means it recruits many more muscles and you get more adaptation and strength much quicker. The dead lift is one of those exercises that makes it really easy for you to see that you're making progress. The weight you're lifting goes up very quickly.

- Stand in front of a barbell with your feet shoulder-width apart and your toes pointing forward. Focus directly ahead of you.
- Arrange one hand with an overhand grip and one with an underhand grip.
- With a neutral back and neck, bend down and pick up the bar and return to the standing position, with the bar gently touching the middle of your thighs. You should be leaning back very slightly.
- Take the bar back to mid-shin or the floor, depending on your ability and range of movement.

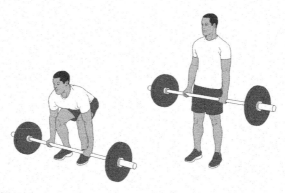

BENCH PRESS

You've pulled with the dead lift and now you're going to switch muscle groups and push with some bench-pressing. This allows you to work multiple large muscle groups, such as chest and shoulders, and stabilizing muscles such as triceps. It's also easy to mess around with – you can change the angle, the tempo and grip position, as well as rep range. Don't try to lift weights that are out of your range because there's no point doing bad form and bad reps that will inevitably end in injury.

- You'll need a training buddy to act as your spotter (or ask someone in the gym to help you). Alternatively, you can use a Smith machine – a weight-training machine with a barbell fixed within steel rails – which allows you to perform exercises safely when training on your own, as you hook the weight on and off.
- Lie back on a flat bench. Either place your feet flat on the bench or on either side of the bench on the floor.
- Take the bar with your hands positioned just over shoulder-width apart. You should be helped with the first part of the exercise, especially when there's a lot of weight on the bar.
- Slowly lower the bar to your chest.
- Explode back to the start position with your elbows locked out or straight.

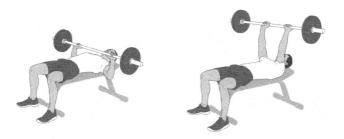

PULL-UPS

This is a great exercise for building mass and strength. You feel your own bodyweight and use your pure natural strength to pull yourself up and over.

- Using an overhand grip, put your hands on the pull-up bar just over shoulder-width apart.
- Cross your ankles and raise your heels until they are at a 90-degree angle – this will stop you from rocking around and ensure you engage the right muscles.
- Pull yourself up until your chin is slightly above the bar. Return to the start position.
- If you struggle with this exercise, add a resistance band under your feet, which will act as a counterbalance, so you're no longer lifting all of your bodyweight.
- Alternatively, you could put a bench or a chair beneath the pull-up bar, which will enable you to jump up before you slowly let yourself down.

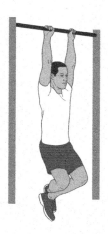 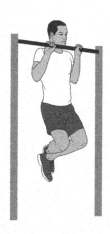

BODYWEIGHT DIPS

Like the traditional pull-up, this is a great barometer of strength. There is no better feeling than being able to dip your own bodyweight repetitively.

- Jump onto the dip bars with your elbows locked or straight behind you, your ankles crossed, your legs at 90 degrees and your chest high.
- Focus in front of you as you lower your body down until your elbows are at 90 degrees.
- Return to the original position.
- You can add resistance by holding a dumbbell or a plate between your legs.

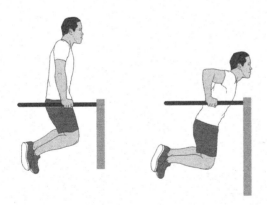

SQUATS

Developing muscle mass on your legs is tough. You're going to have to go through some pain when you're in the gym, and then your legs will possibly be sore for several days afterwards. I believe that training your legs also helps you to transform your upper body. That's because there will be a big chemical response, which will help you to build muscle tissue pretty much everywhere.

- Try to use a neck pad as that adds some comfort.
- Stand in front of an Olympic bar in a squat rack or cage, which should be around shoulder height.
- With your feet shoulder-width apart, lift the bar off carefully and take two steps back while still focusing forward.
- Point your toes slightly outwards. Squat down, so sticking your glutes or bottom out, until your knees are at 90 degrees.
- Pause and return to the start position.

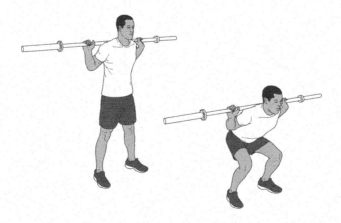

CHRIS'S WORKOUT

Dead lift x 25 reps

Cardio

Dead lift x 20 reps

Bench press x 20 reps

Cardio

Dead lift x 15 reps

Bench press x 15 reps

Pull-ups x 15 reps

Cardio

Dead lift x 10 reps

Bench press x 10 reps

Pull-ups x 10 reps

Bodyweight dips x 10 reps

Cardio

Dead lift x 8 reps

Bench press x 8 reps

Pull-ups x 8 reps

Bodyweight dips x 8 reps

Squats x 8 reps

Cardio

JOHN BOYEGA
FOR STAR WARS

H

At the start of training, like a lot of people, John wasn't naturally coordinated, but it didn't faze him. He was happy to just **GIVE EVERYTHING A GO** and I think that's amazing. When you're a beginner, or starting a new programme, you can feel a little self-conscious in the gym. But even though you may not have great strength or coordination yet, you're **ON THE RIGHT PATH** to feeling good and your confidence will only grow as you improve.

I taught John to **LIVE IN THE MOMENT** with his training rather than always fast-forwarding in his mind to what he was doing next. If you're not completely focused on the present, you won't be concentrating on having **GOOD FORM**, which is absolutely key to avoiding injury and building performance.

Shooting a Star Wars movie comes with unprecedented challenges. There tends to be many intricately choreographed fight scenes, which actors do while wearing bulky costumes that make movement challenging. John Boyega had to move as though he had been trained as a stormtrooper. That was key to preparing him for his role in two of the three Star Wars movies he starred in, *The Last Jedi* and *The Rise of Skywalker*. I designed a programme that would give him the speed, agility and endurance that he needed to portray Finn, and to make it seem as though his fight scenes were almost effortless.

When John came to me, he wasn't in amazing shape, but it wasn't all bad. I just felt as though he hadn't been on the right programme nor had the right focus. I find that lots of young actors are preoccupied with lifting and becoming bigger, rather than thinking about what kind of fitness they need for their roles and to perform the stunts involved effectively.

I changed John's programme around a bit, though still using some similar conditioning techniques and integrating them within my go-to 5–2 method. That changes how the body responds because you're not just focused on developing muscle tissue, but also on maintaining existing muscle tissue while reducing body fat. You're also enhancing your movement, which is exactly what John and I thought he needed for the role.

I have often said to John and other actors I have trained, 'This is how much time we've got for this workout. Lock the door. This is now your environment. No one is coming in to disturb you.' If I am training an actor, and I've left the gym door open, nine times out of ten, someone will come in and disturb us. You might be in the middle of an exercise and a person will enter and say they've got a quick question (it is never quick). That's enormously frustrating for me because I need complete concentration if an actor is going to stay in the present and maintain a high level of intensity. You should also try to minimize disruptions to your workout. Be in your zone.

ACTIVATION AND CARDIO

I would often set up an activation agility circuit in the gym for John. Typically, the activation would be multidirectional, preparing muscles for action. I liked to use exercises such as slaloming in and out of cones, a fast-feet ladder run and a plyometric jump. That was followed by some kind of sprint with deceleration drills, as well as running backwards. Then we would do a push drill, sometimes with a sled (a simple sled-like device which you can load with weights then push and pull), as well as resistance band work. In between most of these drills there would be some form of dynamic stretching. Activation and warm-up would normally take about fifteen minutes. For cardio John liked pad work, but I encouraged him to do ladder work as I knew that would give him the fast feet he needed for the movie. Around 50 to 60 per cent of all running injuries are from deceleration, as we have taught ourselves to accelerate but not to slow down. Ask yourself this: when was the last time you ran backwards? Train your brakes and put yourself in reverse.

JOHN'S 5–2 WORKOUT

LOW CABLE CHEST PRESS

I used a lot of cables with John as he preferred them over dumbbells and we decided they were just as effective. I was also happy because cables allow you to recruit many secondary stabilizing groups, so you're working out primary and supportive muscle groups. In this exercise, the primary muscle group, the chest, is stabilized through the shoulders, and you're also using the arms.

- With your back facing the cable machine, take an overhand grip on the low cables.
- Take three steps and move away with your arms in a retracted position.
- Bring one foot forward. Then, with a neutral back and with your chest up slightly and the palms of your hands facing you, bring the cables up until they are level with your forehead.
- Squeeze, hold for three seconds and then return to the start position.

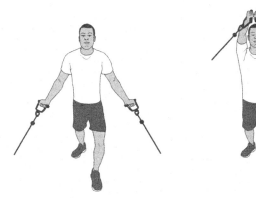

HIGH CABLE CHEST PRESS

By doing a low cable and then a high cable, you're creating variation in the sequence in which the muscle fibres fire. The whole muscle group is used, but this type of variation ensures you're shifting emphasis in the fibre firing sequence.

- Move the cables up above your head and grasp them with your hands.
- Step forward and slightly away from the cable machine with your chest up high, this time bringing the cables low until your palms meet in front of your body (around waist height).
- Squeeze for three seconds and allow the cables to return to their original position.

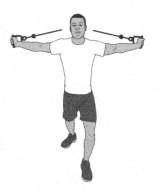
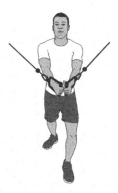

LOW CABLE WOOD CHOP

This is another exercise that uses multiple muscle groups and plenty of movement. You're working the glutes, obliques and all the main core muscles, as well as your arms. As you're using these muscle groups, you're raising your heart rate, which makes it quite cardiovascular.

- Standing side on to the cable, with the cable in a low position, grasp the handle with both hands. Your arms are across your body.
- Take two steps away from the pulley.
- Lean down and bend the leg that is closest to the pulley while straightening the other leg.
- Explode through the glutes, quads and the core, and then use your straight arms to bring the pulley across your body at a 45-degree angle.
- Your eyes should always follow your hands – that's key with this exercise.
- Repeat on the other side.

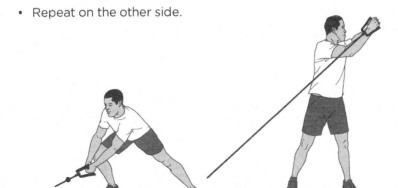

ARM MATRIX

This matrix is great for bicep and forearm development, and with the final exercise you're also training a small muscle in your shoulder, teres minor, which gives you good posture and prevents your shoulders from rolling forward.

- This can be performed either kneeling, standing or sitting on a bench.
- The first exercise is double dumbbell bicep curls. The dumbbells should be about 6 inches away from your legs facing outwards. Slowly raise your dumbbells up to shoulder height.
- Lift your elbows a couple of inches higher for extra pressure and then return to the start position.
- Change the hand position so that your palms are now facing your body and the dumbbells are close to your legs.
- Curling the dumbbells up to shoulder height and then with a little tip of the elbows, return to the start position. This changes the emphasis on the part of the bicep you're training.

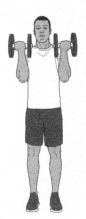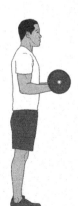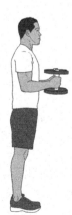

- Maintaining the intensity, raise the dumbbells up, with your palms now facing upwards towards the ceiling. The dumbbells are touching each other in front of you. This is a medial and lateral rotation.
- Keep your elbows tight by your side and push the dumbbells up and away from each other until they are about 10 or 15 inches apart.
- Return to the start position.

SHOULDER MATRIX

I like to use a matrix of shoulder exercises as that allows you to target each part of the shoulder in turn.

- Start with a pair of dumbbells out in front of you at waist height with your arms slightly bent.
- Raise the dumbbells out to the side to shoulder height, maintaining a slight bend in the elbow, keeping the emphasis on the muscle and not on the joint.
- Return to the start position.
- Turn the dumbbells so your palms are facing your body. With a slightly bent elbow, raise one of the dumbbells in front of you to shoulder height.
- Return to the start position. Then repeat using the other arm.
- Then bring the dumbbells up so they are almost resting on your shoulders.
- Press them above your head so you are touching them gently together, then return to the start position.
- For the fourth and final part of the matrix, bend over with a neutral back, with the dumbbells hanging in front of you, just below the chest.

- Using a reverse motion, bring the dumbbells away from your body with slightly bent elbows. You will feel your upper back pinch together. Squeeze and then return the dumbbells to the original position.

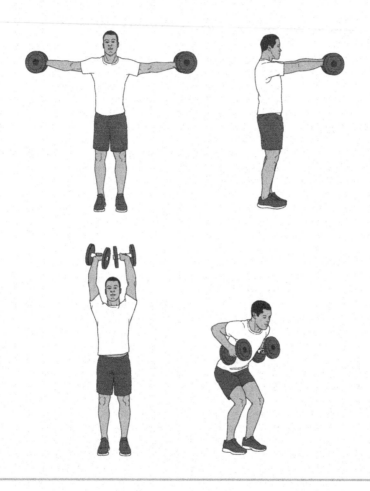

JOHN'S WORKOUT

Low cable chest press x 25 reps

Cardio

Low cable chest press x 20 reps

High cable chest press x 20 reps

Cardio

Low cable chest press x 15 reps

High cable chest press x 15 reps

Low cable wood chop x 15 reps on both sides

Cardio

Low cable chest press x 10 reps

High cable chest press x 10 reps

Low cable wood chop x 10 reps on both sides

Arm matrix x 10 reps

Cardio

Low cable chest press x 8 reps

High cable chest press x 8 reps

Low cable wood chop x 8 reps on both sides

Arm matrix x 8 reps

Shoulder matrix x 8 reps

Cardio

7 | DON'T BE TOO HARD ON YOURSELF

When you work as closely with actors as I do, you can often see when the pressure of a big role is getting to them. Physically and mentally, making an action movie is a complex process. Some actors perform better under pressure, producing their best work and performances, but it's often a tricky road to get there.

I often use various techniques in my programmes to try to help alleviate this pressure a little. Every other person on the set is demanding something from the actors, but I like to provide for them as much as possible in the form of workouts, recovery and nutrition, as well as some escapism. I don't want the time I spend with clients to feel like work to them; it should seem more like leisure and reward time. Unless it's essential or relevant, I try not to bring work stresses into the gym. When I was with Daniel Craig, I would always try to steer our conversations towards football or rugby or what happened at the weekend, or anything that made us laugh.

It's very easy for actors to get mentally fatigued before they're physically tired. They're trying to embody a character – they might have a lot of dialogue to remember, or a particular accent or mannerism to master. That can be exhausting. They're always aiming for perfection, and not just with the physical element of their roles. On every film, once shooting begins, the hardest part of my job is knowing when to say to an actor that rest is going to be more beneficial than working out.

Adam Driver is ex-military. As I'm also a former military man, I understood the ex-marine's intensity and regimented mentality that he brought to the gym when I was training him for *Star Wars*. I saw how dedicated he was when preparing for his role. But occasionally we would push each other too hard during our 4.30 a.m. workouts at the gym in Ireland, where some of the film was being shot. There were occasions when I had to tell Adam that enough was enough. I would say to him, 'Let's do our recovery session now.' But I knew that in his mind he wanted to push himself even harder and keep going. Persuading someone not to train is sometimes more difficult than encouraging and motivating someone to work out. Adam wanted to exercise for one or two hours in the gym every day, regardless of how he was feeling or how busy his schedule was, and I often had to talk him out of it. Sometimes it's not how hard you work, but how hard you recover.

Actors sometimes have to go to quite a dark place in their minds to portray a character, and this can take its toll during a shoot. When I'm training an actor for a major transformation, I like to micro-manage every aspect of the process to make sure they don't get ill. I'm constantly monitoring how they're looking, feeling and responding.

I also ensure they don't do anything to put their health at risk, which in the long term could be hard to come back from. You should always be able to revert to your original state. It can be tricky when an actor has to lose weight for a role, as inevitably they start to enjoy the feeling of being lighter. But usually that only lasts for a certain amount of time, and they will then begin to get fatigued and the body can start breaking down in a way that's irreparable. Never compromise your long-term health for short-term benefits; it's just not worth it.

Perhaps you have a tendency to work too hard in pursuit of

your fitness objectives? You should always avoid pushing yourself to an extreme in your life. It's not healthy for your body or your brain.

Sometimes we put ourselves under too much pressure to reach particular goals, or give ourselves a hard time and then end up tiring ourselves out mentally. It's possible to become so mentally exhausted that you're incapable of doing anything physical that will allow you to get to where you want to be. Know that mental fatigue will stop you before physical fatigue does; it's your brain that tells your body to stop, not the other way around. You must look after your brain in exactly the same way that you look after your body if you are to enjoy the best mental and physical health.

I also always talk to my clients about not being hard on themselves; accept that there are going to be days when you lack motivation and you're not going to be up for a full, intense workout. In fact, you can use those days in other ways that are beneficial. You don't always have to push, because sometimes that's just not possible.

MENTAL WELLBEING COMES FIRST

Your mental health and wellbeing should be your absolute priority, rather than how you think you look in the mirror. If you feel good, you're going to look good, as that's only going to help bring out your confidence, energy and general zest for life.

It's easy to become solely interested in your aesthetic, as that will initially give your ego a boost when others congratulate you on how much weight you've lost or how much muscle you've gained. But that's not as important as how you feel about yourself on the inside. I think the best compliment that people can ever pay you is that they want to spend time with you because you're a fun, positive person. We're so used to being impressed by the visual appearance, but it would be amazing if we started praising each other more about feelings and positivity.

The pressures of social media put even more of our focus on the aesthetic, and it's important not to get wrapped up in this often unrealistic portrayal of what it means to be fit and healthy. These accounts are often full of people who care more about their external appearance than anything else, and will do whatever it takes to reach what they see as perfection; pills, potions and filters are not the way to performance, or a recipe for good mental health. If you're compromising your mental health in the pursuit of extreme or quick-fix solutions, that's going to eventually catch up with you.

Allow your brain and body to help and complement each other; if you feel good in your head, then you'll pay more attention to your body, and when you feel good in your body, you'll be so much happier. When you're in a positive place mentally, you're very aware that you can actively push yourself to get results. And then when you think you've achieved those physical results, the boost gives you that sense of euphoria. If you get it right, it can be a virtuous circle, with the brain and the body being catalysts for each other. They're feeding off each other's positivity.

When I first started training Sam Worthington for *Wrath of the Titans*, exercise wasn't his priority. When I met him, he didn't have a great relationship with working out and nutrition. Although he would exercise, his heart wasn't in it, and I think that was because he thought training for a movie meant taking the old-school approach of doing arduous workouts to the point of being unable to breathe and then later collapsing from exhaustion on the sofa.

As I told Sam, exercising should re-energize you. After you've finished, you should experience that endorphin rush and feel as though you've set yourself up for a great day. You shouldn't feel like you want to go back to bed or lie down on the sofa. That is a big indication that your balance is off. You should have stimulated your brain to be more efficient and more alert, and all your senses should be heightened. That's the whole wellbeing package.

NO SUCH THING AS A BAD DAY

Sometimes it's not possible to accomplish everything you want to every day, or to work out at full intensity all the time. But instead of stressing out about that, try telling yourself that there's no such thing as a bad day, think about what you have actually achieved and start looking forward to the next session. I take the view that as long as you have done something rather than nothing, and that might just be fifteen minutes of cardio or stretching, you will have a good sense of wellbeing for the day. When I was younger, I used to be hard on myself if I missed a workout, but I learned not to give myself a hard time and turn it into a positive.

Fitness is probably the only part of your day where failure can be a positive. When you've exhausted yourself and you have trained to failure – which is when the muscle is so fatigued it can't do another rep – the brain recognizes this and says: 'I don't want to feel like this again. I'm going to do everything physically and mentally to create that adaption so when these stresses are put on me again, I can cope.' That's why failure is a positive. Adaptation will see you get stronger and faster. When anyone says to me during a workout, 'I failed, I can't do it,' I reply, 'That's great, that's what I wanted to happen.' Don't beat yourself up about your fitness failures; you should be welcoming them.

It takes a while to adapt to this mindset, but bodybuilders have been doing it for years. Failure can often be a goal. But don't make it your target in every session, as sometimes you want to complete workouts and to feel as though your sessions are becoming easier and less stressful. That's when you notice your progression.

SOMETIMES LESS IS MORE

If it seems as though you're no longer progressing, it might not be because you're not working hard enough. Instead, it could be that you're working too hard or without enough diversity, or you're simply not giving your body enough time to recover. When your results start to plateau, maybe consider taking a short break rather than increasing the time and intensity of your workouts. Or you could go into your active recovery mode, which is when you switch your mindset from progression to recovery and relaxation, while still staying active.

There is no point upping the intensity, weights or reps to unrealistically chase your goals, as that will result in compounded fatigue, which is fatigue on top of fatigue on top of fatigue. Listen to your body, as it's always going to tell you what it wants and needs.

It's inevitable that at the beginning of our fitness programmes we can start to see some pretty dramatic results – that might be a visual change in our body composition, strength gains or more energy. But we always want a little bit more, so we push ourselves to try to get those additional improvements. But what often happens is that you don't get the same results as those in the first few weeks, and this can be disheartening. My advice is to stick with the programme. Don't change anything. Allow yourself to feel fitter, let the workouts become easier. Why make things tougher when you can get exactly the same results and progress by taking the more sustainable route?

I think most of us imagine that the harder we push ourselves the more progress we're going to make. A lot of the time, that's not the case. One of the worst mistakes you can make is to deprive yourself of nutrition or start getting up earlier to do longer sessions. If you stick to your routine, and allow yourself to feel progression, perhaps over an extended period, that's more likely to give you your gains over the long term. It's a much more sustainable mindset with which to approach your fitness.

One sign I look out for when lifting weights, for example – and this is a great indicator that enough is enough – is when your muscle goes from a hard, pumped and functional state into a soft and unresponsive condition. You can't get any blood into the muscle and that's because it's exhausted.

THE TEN-MINUTE MENTAL-HEALTH CHECK

Most people at some time find that everything's a struggle and they don't have the energy or motivation to work out. Life can take over and intrude on our training. Everyone has their vulnerabilities. I think we all have days when we're lacking motivation. Being aware of that should stop you from being hard on yourself. Don't imagine for one minute that everyone else is always motivated and energized all of the time. They're not.

At the start of most workouts with clients, I'll spend a few minutes understanding where their energy and motivation levels are. I normally begin by asking them how they slept, because if you've had a poor sleep then that has a huge impact on how energized you are going to be feeling about working out. I also give them the opportunity to offload any stresses, as these have an effect on their energy levels and how I'm going to structure the intensity of the workout.

You need to have a similar conversation with yourself. Before you train, find the time and space to give yourself a quick mental-health check. Ask yourself: 'How am I functioning? Are all my senses as responsive as they're supposed to be? How are my concentration levels?' You're assessing how you're feeling and the intensity at which you're ready to train. You can do this during your activation. Or you could do it separately when you're sitting down in a more meditative way. Allow around ten minutes to go through your mental checklist and assess whether you're in a good place. We're all so externally focused. We're always looking outwards, but you need to turn that around and focus inwards, and be in tune with your wellbeing, with your brain, breathing, heart rate, anxiety and stress. You might simply ask: 'How am I coping today?'

I find that a good question to consider is whether you're mentally aware of being in the moment. I think we're either thinking about what's going to happen in the future, or we're going over what has occurred in the past. We rarely, if ever, sit in the present, and that's such an important thing to do. Focus on yourself right here in this moment. You want to be able to say to yourself: 'Yes, I'm functioning, my heart rate feels good, my breathing is controlled, and my body feels strong and responsive.' Ask yourself about your sleep and what you've been eating. How's your nutrition making you feel? Food is so emotional. Are you enjoying it? Or are you resenting it?

You should have a checklist of everything you want to achieve, and you should ask yourself whether each of the elements of your programme – training, recovery, nutrition – are all where you want them to be. Assess how motivated you are feeling today. If you had to rate your physical and mental state between one and ten, what score would you give yourself?

Ultimately, you want to reach a stage where you do this almost unconsciously. Whatever helps you to have good mental strength and stamina is going to help you physically.

ADAPTING TO YOUR MENTAL STATE

This is never about allowing yourself to be lazy but about finding a compromise, and understanding that sometimes life stops you from training at the intensity you want to. You'll soon learn the difference between laziness and genuine mental and physical fatigue. By asking the questions I just suggested, you can learn to distinguish between the two. Accept that things happen which can alter our moods. Maybe you didn't eat well the night before, or perhaps you've just had an argument with a friend or a family member, and that's drained you of your desire to visit the gym or go for a run or do whatever you had been planning to do.

Remember that you should always try to do something to ensure you're making progress, but you don't always have to go all-out every day as that will lead to burnout. To avoid that, you need to listen to your mind and body, and don't put yourself under too much stress. Always try to start and end on a positive.

Say to yourself before a session: 'I will do this.' And then tell yourself at the end: 'I have done this.' Then you will have a sense of achievement.

There are going to be days when you have lots of natural energy, or even synthetic stimulation from a double espresso, and you feel amazing. That's the time to turn the intensity up. Make the most of feeling like that. But on the days when you're not feeling your best, turn the intensity down and don't worry about it.

Depending on what people tell me about their sleep and energy levels, I adjust the session. I always have a twenty-minute, a forty-minute and a sixty-minute workout in my head, and I'll give them the one that I think is the most appropriate, based on the answers to my questions. You can do the same – if you feel as though you can't manage the full session you had been planning, give yourself a lighter day and do twenty or forty minutes instead.

Be honest with yourself as that will help you to avoid setbacks. If you've had interrupted sleep, you could reduce the intensity as well as the time – bring everything down by 10, 15 or 20 per cent of what your perceived optimum is. Just stay flexible.

I felt like I learned the most about mental fatigue from training Ralph Fiennes while he was working in the theatre. Theatre requires much more concentration than shooting a film because of the pressures involved in getting it right first time. You can't reset and go again. I learned from Ralph the distinct difference between mental fatigue and physical fatigue. He showed me how mental fatigue isn't necessarily a sign that you're physically exhausted, and that when your mind is tired your body is still capable of something. Normally in that situation, I would suggest doing something very straightforward and simplistic that you've done before and doesn't take a lot of thought. The last thing you should be trying is anything complex for the first time. You don't want an activity that requires much concentration.

All my programming is extremely flexible. If you give yourself strict parameters to work within, it's going to be tough as it doesn't allow you to adapt your plan based on how you are feeling when you wake up. I don't like people being so regimented in life. It can be stressful because if you don't accomplish certain goals, you won't feel a sense of achievement. Give yourself some flexibility. If you're going to get the best results, you need to be engaged, willing and able to use your fitness intelligence. You shouldn't be training just for the sake of it.

Clients sometimes say to me that they would feel guilty if they didn't work out at 100 per cent every day. Some people perceive that as failure. But if they are fatigued, I'm happy to tell them that we're not going to train today and we'll be resting instead. If that triggers the response of, 'No, I need to work out,' I can adapt the session with a lower intensity, so at least we're doing something. But often we don't train at all. The next day, my clients usually say that they're so pleased that they didn't exercise the day before – they feel a million times better and now they're raring to go.

JUST GET STARTED

I always feel that getting started is the hardest thing, but once you get going you will be able to judge how much energy you have to put into your session. I'm certain that you can convince yourself to get started with anything if you tell yourself that you're just going to do ten minutes to make yourself feel better.

Getting started can ignite your mood. Your brain will soon find out how you are managing and what you are capable of doing today. Your body will probably find the energy it needs, and once you start releasing some endorphins, you'll be off and away. If you're really not enjoying it and the mood doesn't take you, however, just adapt to how you are feeling. Believe me, you don't want to get injured or become ill, as that could mean weeks or even months of setbacks.

SHOULD I STEP ON THE SCALES?

Too much information can be dangerous. That's why I don't tend to advise clients to step on the scales in the morning – or indeed at any time – as the risk is that the number could ruin their mood for the day. We can all be really hard on ourselves when it comes to our weight, worrying that we haven't lost as much as we wanted, or perhaps even added a few pounds somehow. That number then controls everything we do, how we feel about eating and about food, and it can lead to some extreme and sometimes harmful behaviour.

Using your weight as a metric is not a true reflection of your health and fitness. Our bodies are changing the whole time – your weight in the morning can be several pounds different to the afternoon – so what does that number actually mean? Think about how hard you've worked and how you feel. You've got to be careful about falling into the trap of believing that you're not making progress or improving, as that can make you feel that you have to train harder, but in actual fact the opposite is often true.

You don't have to chase a number when you can instead judge your progress on how you look or, even better, on how you're feeling. Unless you're a professional athlete, and you need to hit a particular weight and body fat percentage, you should never let a number dictate your mood and mentality. Try to get your head around the fact that muscle weighs more than fat, and bear in mind that muscles form the main shape of your body. Always try to focus on body composition rather than on weight.

BLAKE LIVELY FOR
THE RHYTHM SECTION

H

What I saw with Blake was an **UNCOMPROMISING ATTITUDE** and a willingness to give everything a go – she would always take herself **TO THE LIMIT** while we were training for the film.

Blake also knew her limitations and was willing to be honest about them. She was giving feedback about when to push, when to recover and when enough was enough. There were times when Blake had reached her limits and was **BRAVE ENOUGH TO SAY SO**.

I've got so much respect for how Blake found a way of multitasking, being both a new parent and an action-movie star. On dark, cold and very early mornings in Ireland, where *The Rhythm Section* was being filmed, I would ask her to do some squats as part of her workout. As the mother of a young baby, Blake would sometimes suggest doing those exercises with her child strapped to her chest.

Anyone else might use a kettlebell or a weighted jacket, but if you are a new mum, having your baby in a sling is a good way of adding resistance while working out. Obviously, it's not always safe to do this as you're going to be bouncing around for some of the exercises, but it's a good addition for a few of them. Those were great bonding moments for Blake and her daughter, but they were also productive, with the actor completely dedicated to preparing for the movie.

Together, we decided that her character would look completely capable physically, as her role included swimming in open water, fight scenes and handling a weapon. We would work out at 5 a.m. at the house that she had rented in Dublin and whenever I arrived a bit early, she was always ready to go. Sometimes Blake was so enthusiastic that she would be sitting by the door waiting for me. We trained in that house as I didn't want to take her out of her space and her family dynamic for two or three hours. I prefer someone to multitask rather than cancel a session. When Blake was walking or running on the treadmill, she could still speak to her family and deal with everyday home life.

While Blake is an amazing athlete, training her for the movie was not without its complications and challenges as it was a transformative film – her character, Stephanie, changes on screen as the story develops. In the beginning, she was far from athletic, being emaciated and living in deprivation. But Stephanie eventually becomes an assassin and it was my job to aid that transition. Blake needed fast feet, with movement and speed, as well as endurance and hand–eye coordination. She did lots of her own stunts for the movie – actors always like to do as much as they're capable of – and some of the fight choreography was extremely challenging. Blake also needed evasive driving skills. It was a hard process because we were constantly altering the workouts and the nutrition to suit the changing requirements of the character portrayal.

This legs workout – which I did with Blake twice a week – is fast and effective. It's great for cardiovascular fitness, as well as strength and flexibility.

ACTIVATION AND CARDIO

Before any strenuous activity, I like to start with some light activation, preparing the body and the brain to engage with one another, and readying them for work. With Blake that would involve movement-based drills, such as ladder work, some light boxing when she would punch the pads I was holding, and explosive, powerful movements known as plyometrics. I would also get Blake to do something before stunt training or before a specific scene that required dynamic movement, which helped to trigger her aggression and mentally prepare her to portray the character. For cardio, Blake would do incline walking on the treadmill while wearing a weighted vest, along with a sprinkling of sprints.

BLAKE'S 5–2 WORKOUT

SQUATS

Depending on Blake's energy levels that day, I could turn the volume up and add intensity to these squats, or I could turn it down by making it more simplistic.

- Stand with your feet just over shoulder-width apart and your toes pointing slightly outwards.
- Lower yourself until your knees are at a 90-degree angle and hold for a count of four.
- Explode back through your heels to return to the start position.
- For variation, adapt the squat by holding a medicine ball above your head. Or you could combine a squat with a sidestep: sidestep, then a squat, and repeat.

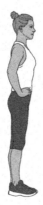
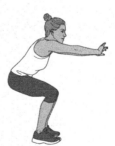

LADDER WORK

This exercise is like a dance – one foot is going to be touching every single square of the ladder with a toe, as fast as you can and with as much momentum and grace as possible. This gives you fast feet and coordinated lower-body movement. Ladder work is cardiovascular – it raises your heart rate – and is also lots of fun.

- Start at one end, just to the left of the ladder with your feet shoulder-width apart.
- Move your right foot about 10 inches into the first space of the ladder, gently touching it with your toe, and then continue along the squares until you reach the end of the ladder.
- Then turn around, standing on the right of the ladder, and return using your left foot. Try to look straight ahead rather than at your feet. You can mix up the speed and tempo.

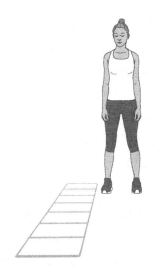
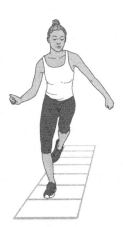

SPLIT SQUAT WITH SHOULDER PRESS

Adding two movements together – in this case a lunge and a shoulder press – creates more intensity and enables you to be more dynamic and coordinated. It gets everything firing at once rather than separately.

- Stand with your feet just over shoulder-width apart, holding a dumbbell in each hand positioned up by your shoulders.
- Lunge forward, dropping your rear leg until your knee kisses the floor.
- Explode upwards, raising the dumbbells up above your head until they gently touch.
- Bring the dumbbells down, lowering your rear leg to the floor again. Do one set with one leg and then swap over.

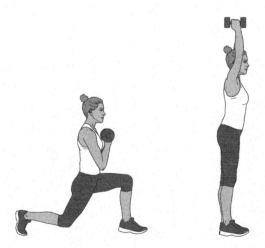

BAND WORK

We're often so linear with our workouts that we sometimes forget about how we can go sideways as well and move around corners. Band work is about being more lateral, and also enhances glute stability. I try to use bands in a matrix form, doing sidesteps as well as forward and backward steps.

- Place one band around your ankles and the second band just over your knees. Your feet are shoulder-width apart and you're bending your legs slightly.
- Clasp your hands in front of you to create energy and focus straight ahead of you.
- Do ten small shuffles to the left and then ten small shuffles to the right.
- For the box step, put your left foot forward around 10 inches until you get tension on the band, and then move your right forward, before moving your left foot back and then your right.

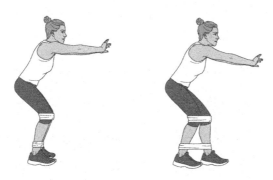

STABILITY WORK

This exercise enhanced Blake's stability and coordination while improving her reflexes.

- If this is new to you, place both feet on the BOSU ball shoulder-width apart. If you make progression with this exercise, try doing it as Blake did: one-legged.
- Engage your glutes and abdominals, and keep your knees soft. Put your hands out in front of you and look up.
- A training partner throws a tennis ball, Pilates ball or weighted beanbag at you in various positions: high to low, and left to right. The throwing directions should be varied, so you're never quite sure where the ball or beanbag will go next.
- After catching and throwing the object back, return to the original position so you're ready for the next throw.

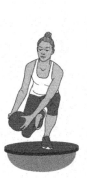 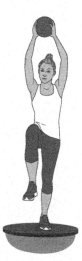

BLAKE'S WORKOUT

Squats x 25 reps

Cardio

Squats x 25 reps
Ladder work x 4 rounds

Cardio

Squats x 25 reps
Ladder work x 4 rounds
Split squat with shoulder press x 10 each leg

Cardio

Squats x 25 reps
Ladder work x 4 rounds
Split squat with shoulder press x 10 each leg
Band work x 15 each side

Cardio

Squats x 25 reps
Ladder work x 4 rounds
Split squat with shoulder press x 10 each leg
Band work x 15 each side
Stability work x 10 reps

Cardio

CHRIS PRATT FOR
GUARDIANS OF THE GALAXY

H

No matter what, and even if he was exhausted, Chris **ALWAYS TURNED UP** for his sessions with me. But he had the ability to **LISTEN TO HIS BODY** and recognize when he was too tired. Chris would walk into the gym and say to me: 'Hey, it's Thursday and it feels as though the week is catching up with me. I always want to do something, but I don't want to do too much today.'

Chris and I got the **BALANCE** just right – he was willing to put in the work, but he wouldn't compromise his health just for the sake of doing a tough session. You can learn from Chris – be aware of what your body is telling you and **NEVER IGNORE THE SIGNS OF FATIGUE**.

Even when they are wearing costumes, actors are exposed on screen. There's nowhere to hide. But they're never more exposed than when they are shirtless, as Chris was for the prison shower scene in the first *Guardians of the Galaxy* film.

When I read that in the script, I marked it and immediately referred to the schedule to find out the date when Chris would be shooting the scene – I needed to know how much time I had to get him ready. That was the moment in the movie when Chris would reveal all the hard work that he had put into his preparations and when I hoped people would say: 'Wow, he really got in amazing shape for that role.'

I assume that when Chris was hired for *Guardians of the Galaxy*, someone on the production team must have had a light-bulb moment and realized what his ultimate potential would be. But it's always a bit of a risk when an actor hasn't been in an athletic role before. But that's why I'm around – to help such actors to achieve their full fitness potential.

When I met Chris for the first time I could see that he was a big guy, but I knew instantly that he had the potential to look immense. He is a truly dedicated athlete. His background as a high-school wrestler gave him the right mentality – he knew what it was going to take. Chris wasn't completely out of shape. There was just some sculpting to be done for his role as Peter Quill, or Star-Lord. Chris wanted to be in the best possible condition and there was no way that wasn't going to happen. He was committed to the vision of his character. You can't develop such a powerful physique unless you are 100 per cent invested. I've since worked with Chris on the Jurassic World movies, which were also very physical. But preparing him for that first *Guardians of the Galaxy* film was the bigger challenge.

Chris and I were always adapting workouts to match his energy levels on any given day. We were forever conscious of not pushing him too hard to prevent him from getting ill or injured. He couldn't risk being so fatigued that he wouldn't recover properly.

ACTIVATION AND CARDIO

As Chris is a big, muscular guy, I wanted him to feel light, dynamic and flexible, and to know that he could function without restrictions. Chris enjoyed doing animalistic movements, such as bear crawls and side crab walks. For cardio, Chris's preference was the rowing machine – he would do a sprint row of 500 or 1,000 metres, depending on the workout. He also skipped and did battle ropes, as well as multidirectional agility drills on the track, such as slaloming between cones, ladder work, mini hurdles, sidesteps, grapevine and sprinting.

CHRIS'S 5–2 WORKOUT

OLYMPIC LIFTS – CLEAN AND JERK

The main reason I got Chris to do this was because it's fun, with lots of movements involved, as well as being a great compound exercise. I don't always use complex exercises such as this with my clients, because they are technical and can require a lot of instruction. But I knew that Chris had the experience of training from his college days, so he was more than capable of doing the clean and jerk. If you have some coordination, you should be able to master this and then the benefits are huge.

- Using a moderate weight, stand in front of the bar with your feet shoulder-width apart.
- Use an overhand grip and keep a neutral back and neck. You can use the mirror to ensure you have good form.
- As you lift the bar up, it will naturally brush your thighs.
- With your elbows high, flip the bar over so that your palms are facing the ceiling.
- Raise the bar until your elbows are locked out or straight.
- Return the bar to your chest and allow it to flip back to your thighs and then back down to the ground.

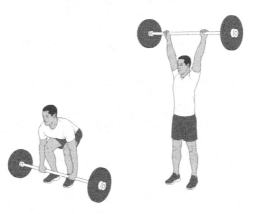

BENCH PRESS

This is the go-to exercise for strength and muscular development. You're hitting multiple muscle groups with an all-round compound exercise that is great for developing the chest, as well as the shoulders and triceps. You can also mix it up with different hand positions and tempo – the variety you can get with this exercise is almost endless, which is great for adaptation.

- You'll need a training buddy to act as your spotter (or ask someone in the gym to help you). Alternatively, you can use a Smith machine to hook a bar on and off for safety.
- Lie back on a flat bench. Either place both feet on the bench or have them on either side of the bench on the floor.
- Take the bar with your hands positioned just over shoulder-width apart.
- You should be helped with the first part of the exercise, especially when there's a lot of weight on the bar.
- Slowly lower the bar to your chest.
- Explode back to the start position with your elbows locked out or straight.

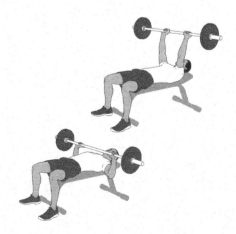

DEAD LIFT

Again, this is brilliant for strength and muscular development, but it's a little more challenging for anyone taller than 6 foot, such as Chris. That's because of the biomechanics – with greater height comes greater distance, and that always creates difficulties when taking something off the floor. I adapted this exercise for Chris by using raised blocks, so he wasn't picking the bar up directly off the ground – this allowed us to really load the bar with weights.

- Stand in front of a barbell with your feet shoulder-width apart and your toes pointing forward. Focus directly ahead of you.
- Arrange one hand with an overhand grip and one with an underhand grip. This gives you more power and control.
- With a neutral back and neck, bend down and pick up the bar and return to the standing position, with the bar gently touching the middle of your thighs. Lean back very slightly.
- Take the bar back to mid-shin or the floor, depending on your ability and range of movement.

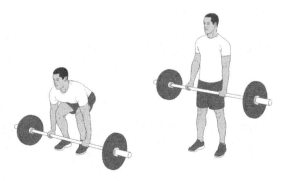

SHOULDER MATRIX

Chris did lateral raises, shoulder press into forward raises, then bent-over rows. This provides you with strength and stability, as well as definition.

- For the lateral raises, raise the dumbbells to the side with slightly bent elbows so they are parallel with your ears.
- Return to the start position and transition from lateral raises into shoulder press. Hold the dumbbells so that your arms are at 90 degrees on either side and the dumbbells are about 6 inches away from your ears.
- Press the dumbbells in the air so they gently kiss each other.
- Come back down so your elbows and arms are at 90 degrees.
- Transition into forward raises. Bring the dumbbells so they are touching your thighs and then lift one dumbbell up with a slightly bent elbow to shoulder height and return to the start position. Repeat on the other side.
- Transition into bent-over row. You need to have a little bit of bend in your knees. Maintain a neutral spine, back and neck. The dumbbells are dangling in front of you below chest height. With a slight bend in your elbows, retract the dumbbells so they are parallel with your shoulders and then return to the start position.

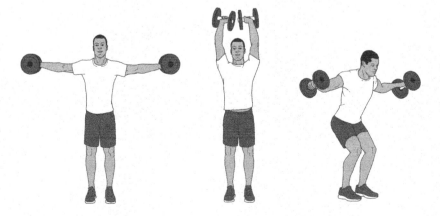

ARM MATRIX

As with the shoulder matrix, I combined several exercises that were completed in quick succession. I like to finish with an arm matrix as I believe the arms are already partially fatigued from previous exercises. Start with normal double bicep curls, before going immediately into pistol curls and then straight into medial/lateral rotations, which are good for posture and forearm development. You then finish off with regular tricep dips with your feet raised. Feel free to add resistance.

- Start off with the dumbbells beside your thighs. Keep your elbows tucked in and push the hands a little bit away so they are about 10 inches from your thighs. You can do this standing up or sitting down.
- Bring the dumbbells up with your palms facing towards the ceiling.
- Return to the start position with an even tempo.
- Keep the dumbbells in the same position, but move your hands so they are now facing you and the dumbbells are tight to your side. Bring the dumbbells up to shoulder height and then return to the start position beside your thighs.

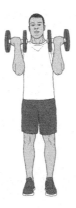 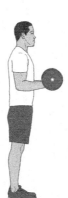 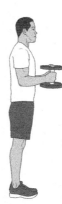

- Transition into medial rotation. Bring the dumbbells up so your arms are at 90 degrees.
- Turn so your palms are facing the ceiling. Kiss the dumbbells gently together and then move them away from each other about 10 to 15 inches.
- Bring the dumbbells back down.
- As you transition out of that, you're going to need a bench for the tricep dips. For added resistance, use two benches and raise your legs. You should be almost sitting on your hands, with your fingers coming off the edge of the bench.
- Lower yourself down until your elbows are at 90 degrees. Return to the start position.
- To add more intensity, look up at the ceiling and lock out or straighten your elbows, pause for three seconds and then restart the exercise.

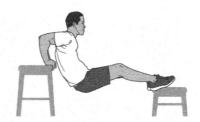

CHRIS'S WORKOUT

Olympic lifts – clean and jerk x 25 reps

Cardio

Olympic lifts – clean and jerk x 20 reps
Bench press x 20 reps

Cardio

Olympic lifts – clean and jerk x 15 reps
Bench press x 15 reps
Dead lift x 15 reps

Cardio

Olympic lifts – clean and jerk x 10 reps
Bench press x 10 reps
Dead lift x 10 reps
Shoulder matrix x 10 reps

Cardio

Olympic lifts – clean and jerk x 8 reps
Bench press x 8 reps
Dead lift x 8 reps
Shoulder matrix x 8 reps
Arm matrix x 8 reps

Cardio

JAKE GYLLENHAAL FOR
PRINCE OF PERSIA

H

We can all learn from Jake's **METICULOUS** approach
to fitness. I loved how he took everything to the **NEXT
LEVEL**. For example, he never wanted to act tired or
out of breath – instead, he wanted to actually be in
that state, so it looked more authentic. Before those
scenes, I would stand behind the camera and he
would do two or three minutes on the pads.
As they started rolling, he had real sweat running
down his face.

Jake would do these **AMAZING 3.30 A.M. WORKOUTS**; once
we were in the car, he took the opportunity to have an
athlete's nap so he would be ready for the day on set.
He's **A GREAT EXAMPLE** of someone who adapts his day
to achieve his goals.

Most mornings, Jake and I would work out at 3.30 a.m. I've done some early training sessions with actors during my time in the film industry, but never any earlier than the ones I did with Jake. We were on location in Morocco, on the edge of the Sahara, with a ninety-minute drive from the hotel to the set, and Jake had to be there at 6 a.m. That's why we ended up training before the sun came up, with an intensity that most couldn't deal with at any hour.

After a long, full day on set – often more than twelve hours of shooting action scenes in the desert heat – Jake would often run back some of the way through the Sahara Desert, doing around 10 kilometres on the hot sand while I followed in the car. He was happy doing that. I think he found that running in the desert provided a kind of escapism. But once back at the hotel, it was all about recovery, which meant refuelling, hydrating, stretching and sleeping.

'Whatever it takes,' Jake said to me more than once. If you want to be at the top of your game in the film industry, you really have to push yourself if you are going to play physical roles and make them believable. When an actor is physically capable, it allows the audience to buy into their character.

The movie is based on a video game, and I took some references from that. Inspired by how his character moved in the game, Jake had to be able to jump and be extremely agile, like he was doing parkour. He was sprinting everywhere, bouncing around and doing most of his own stunts. There were scenes involving riding horses, which he had to master, as well as choreographed sword fights – and they used heavy swords rather than faking it with lightweight ones. Jake also had to look muscular and capable – he was wearing armour in every scene, but it was sleeveless, so his arms were on show. As long as he stayed hydrated, which he did, I knew that Jake was ready for almost anything. I think we nailed Jake's preparations for the movie.

Jake was invested. He had to put his trust in me. As it was an athletic, strength-based role, that was our primary focus with the workout. We stuck to the big, simple, compound exercises that recruited multiple muscle groups.

ACTIVATION AND CARDIO

Jake liked to sit on the bike and flush his legs through in preparation for the day. For cardio, I got Jake to skip, which was great for hand–eye coordination and rhythm. He would also do two minutes of plyometrics.

JAKE'S 5–2 WORKOUT

BENCH PRESS

This was a major compound exercise to develop upper-body strength, especially around the chest and shoulders. This was particularly important for Jake, as it made his character look more authentic.

- You'll need a training buddy to act as your spotter (or ask someone in the gym to help you). Alternatively, you can use a Smith machine to hook a bar on and off for safety.
- Lie back on a flat bench. Either place both feet on the bench or have them on either side of the bench on the floor.
- Take the bar with your hands positioned just over shoulder-width apart.
- You should be helped with the first part of the exercise, especially when there's a lot of weight on the bar.
- Slowly lower the bar to your chest.
- Explode back to the start position with your elbows locked out or straight.

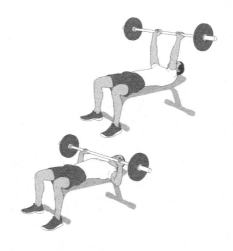

BICEP MATRIX

Using a combination of exercises, with one following immediately after another, creates intensity. This is great for development and definition, as well as thickening fast-twitch and slow-twitch muscle fibres, as you're using weight plus endurance.

- The bicep matrix can be performed either kneeling, standing or sitting on a bench.
- The first exercise is double dumbbell bicep curls. The dumbbells should be about 6 inches away from your legs facing outwards. Slowly raise your dumbbells up to shoulder height.
- Lift your elbows a couple of inches higher for extra intensity and then return to the start position.
- Change the hand position so that your palms are now facing your body and the dumbbells are close to your legs.
- Curling the dumbbells up to shoulder height and then with a little tip of the elbows, return to the start position.
- Maintaining the intensity, raise the dumbbells up, with your palms now facing upwards towards the ceiling. The dumbbells are touching each other in front of you.
- Keep your elbows tight by your side and push the dumbbells up and away from each other until they are about 10 or 15 inches apart.
- Return to the start position.

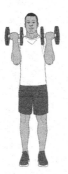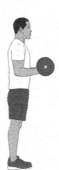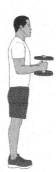

SHOULDER MATRIX

This uses every area of the shoulder. The lateral raises add great definition, the dumbbell press gives you power, and by doing the front portion and the rear portion you're going to get well-balanced shoulder stability.

* For the first exercise, the lateral raises, raise the dumbbells to the side with slightly bent elbows so they are parallel with your ears or the tops of your shoulders.
* Return to the start position and transition from lateral raises into dumbbell press. Hold the dumbbells so that your arms are at 90 degrees on either side and the dumbbells are about 6 inches away from your ears. Press the dumbbells in the air so they gently kiss each other.
* Come back down so your elbows and arms are at 90 degrees.
* Transition into forward raises. Bring the dumbbells so they are touching your thighs.
* Lift one dumbbell up with a slightly bent elbow to shoulder height and return to the start position. Repeat on the other side.
* Transition into bent-over row. You need to have a little bit of bend in your knees. The dumbbells are dangling in front of you below chest height.
* With a slight bend in your elbows, retract the dumbbells so they are parallel with your shoulders and then return to the start position.

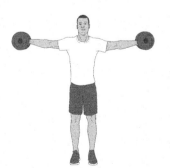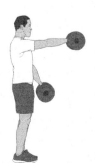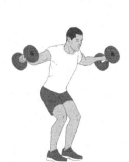

WEIGHTED LUNGES

This is a great way of training the power unit of the body – your glutes. All your speed and strength is initially generated through the glutes. I generally find that men ignore the glutes and women overtrain them. You need to find a balance.

- Stand with your feet shoulder-width apart holding two dumbbells, one on either side of you so they are dangling, with your arms just acting as hooks.
- Take a medium step forward, keeping your feet shoulder width apart. Always ensure that your feet are shoulder-width apart for balance. Lower the rear leg down so the knee either touches the ground or, to make it more comfortable, put a foam block under your knee.
- Drive and power through the front heel so that all the tension goes through the glute. Go down so the knee is at 90 degrees.
- Return to the start position.
- Stay on the same leg to create intensity with the reps, and then change and do the other side.

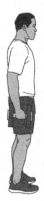
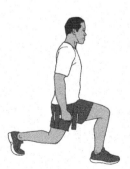

WEIGHTED CORE MATRIX

This is about working around the core, which includes the obliques, abdominals and lower back. I like to mix up the angles, resistance, tempo and tensions.

- Start off lying on the ground with a medicine ball which suits your resistance capability. Hold the ball behind your head with both hands.
- Move the ball with straight arms until it touches your raised knees and you feel your abdominals under tension. Return to the start position.

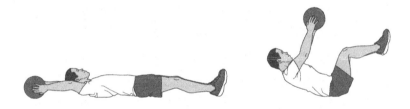

- Immediately go into Russian twists. Sit on the mat, holding a resistance item – this could be a medicine ball, kettlebell, dumbbell or plate – with your legs in front of you at a 45-degree angle and your ankles crossed.

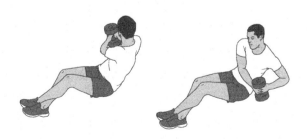

- Lift your legs 6 inches off the ground. Twist to the left, moving the resistance item so it touches the floor, and then return to the start position.
- Twist to the right and lower the item until it touches the floor on that side.
- Transition into leg raises. Lie on your back and move your legs up to 90 degrees and then slowly come back down to 6 inches off the floor. Keep your abdominals tight and engaged, with your lower back engaged and pressed into the ground.

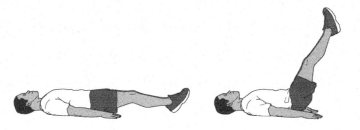

- Move to your knees for this next one: side obliques weighted crunches. Hold a moderate-to-heavy weight in one hand and put one hand behind your head.
- Lower the dumbbell so it just touches the ground, move across to the other side, going past the start position.

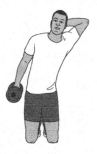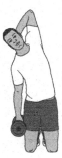

JAKE'S WORKOUT

Bench press x 25 reps

Cardio

Bench press x 20 reps
Bicep matrix x 20 reps

Cardio

Bench press x 15 reps
Bicep matrix x 15 reps
Shoulder matrix x 15 reps

Cardio

Bench press x 10 reps
Bicep matrix x 10 reps
Shoulder matrix x 10 reps
Weighted lunges x 10 reps on each leg

Cardio

Bench press x 8 reps
Bicep matrix x 8 reps
Shoulder matrix x 8 reps
Weighted lunges x 8 reps on each leg
Weighted core matrix x 8 reps

Cardio

ADAM DRIVER FOR STAR WARS

H

Adam Driver is **RELENTLESS**. I think that mentality stems from his time in the military. He understands **INTENSITY AND WORKLOAD** and what it takes to perform a particular way.

You have to completely understand what you're dedicating yourself to because otherwise there's no point. If an actor is doing a big movie transformation, as the trainer you're essentially messing around with their health, and so they must have faith in you. Adam trusted in my plan and believed in me, which is why he was **TOTALLY COMMITTED**. Anyone who is starting a new programme needs to understand what they are embarking on.

If you ever find yourself getting into lightsabre fights with your kids, this could be the workout for you. It's also ideal if you just want to enhance your overall fitness.

When shooting fight scenes in a Star Wars movie, you need to be super athletic. You're using a lot of your upper body, you're rotating at the hips and you need a great deal of power and strength. You're firing the glutes and the hamstrings while also maintaining stability and coordination. In choreographed fight scenes, you're coordinating your whole body; you're constantly lunging, twisting, turning, moving. Those scenes are hard enough to do when you're practising in the stunt room in loose-fitting gym kit. But then you go to the stage to film and you have to perform at the highest level wearing a restrictive costume. You're also dealing with hot lights, hard flooring and needing to stand on your mark in certain positions, while thinking about the camera angles and the added stress of a few hundred people watching you.

Duelling with lightsabres was one of the reasons why Adam needed to be extremely athletic for his role as Kylo Ren. I trained and looked after Adam through his last two Star Wars movies – *The Last Jedi* and *The Rise of Skywalker* – and this is the workout I used for the latter, which was the most demanding of the two.

There is one scene in particular that sticks in my mind – a water scene that featured Adam emerging from the waves. To film that, he spent two or three days getting soaked through and bitterly cold while suspended up high on a wire and wearing a restrictive costume. Indeed, he had to endure a considerable chunk of time on set flying through the air in a harness. Despite all those challenges, Adam had to be capable of doing what the director asked of him, which was physically very intense.

Whereas Daniel Craig needed to look natural and smooth as he moved on screen as James Bond, Adam's movements were a lot more exaggerated. And, unusually for a Star Wars film, in *The Rise of Skywalker* there was an aesthetic shot which featured

Adam with his top off, so I also had to get him ready for that. Actors are happy to do this type of shot if they think it's relevant to the character, but not just for the sake of it, as the preparation work requires far more intricate training and very tailored nutrition.

Though based at Pinewood Studios, Adam also spent quite a bit of time filming on location in Dingle, a small town in south-west Ireland. During the shoot, we would get up at 4 a.m. and be at the gym by around 4.30 a.m. It was so early that the owners gave us a spare set of keys so we could let ourselves in, have an espresso and then work out until 6 a.m., before Adam began a full day's filming.

For Adam, that espresso shot was a godsend, giving him the stimulation he needed before a workout. The early morning training became part of his routine, the way to mark the start of his working day. His mentality was amazing, and his attention to detail and dedication were second to none.

ACTIVATION AND CARDIO

Activation in the Star Wars gym at Pinewood would consist of running up and down a track. It was similar to a footballer's warm-up: Adam would slalom through cones, doing high knee lifts, heel taps, grapevines and small explosive sprints. We would also play some basketball and have a quick game of table tennis, which was fun and also helped to improve his hand–eye coordination and lateral movement. I can't remember ever winning a game of ping-pong against Adam. For cardio, Adam enjoyed his running – he would go out wearing his headphones and listening to music. He liked the escapism.

ADAM'S 5–2 WORKOUT

DEAD LIFT TO SQUAT THRUST

I like this exercise because it's multifaceted – you're working on your strength and movement, and it also has a cardio element. Movements like this are efficient and reduce the amount of time you need to spend in the gym.

- As if you're about to do a conventional dead lift, approach the 20-kilogram Olympic barbell with your feet shoulder-width apart.
- Using an overhand grip, with a neutral back and neck, and engaging your core, lift the bar from the floor to the standing position.
- Lower the bar back down to the floor.
- With your hands on the floor, jump backwards with both feet, and then explosively move them forward into the original dead-lift position.
- Stand and repeat.

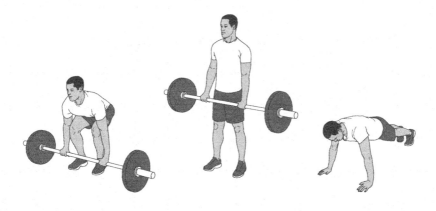

SQUAT THRUST TO PULL-UP

This is another multifaceted exercise that uses strength and agility while raising the heart rate. It's great for creating functional movement patterns, which I knew Adam would need a lot in scenes that involved lunging, getting up off the floor or being in the air.

- As you would for a conventional pull-up, stand underneath the pull-up bar.
- Now squat down with your hands touching the floor.
- Your legs shoot out behind you and then shoot back.
- Using a little bit of momentum, explode upwards and grab the pull-up bar.
- Pull yourself up so your chin is over the bar.
- Lower yourself slightly and then drop to the floor.
- Your hands hit the floor and you're back into the squat.

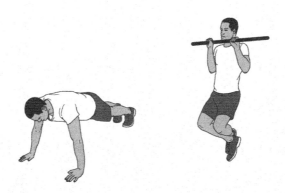

REVERSE LUNGE TO BICEP CURL SEQUENCE

Your glutes are your powerhouse and give you explosive strength. They're the main engine room for power and muscle. This exercise, with its lunge and bicep curl combination, is great for adding glute strength and stability. Like the first two exercises, this one is multifunctional and makes the best use of your time.

- Holding moderate weights – ones with which you can do bicep curls – stand with the dumbbells beside your thighs, with your feet shoulder-width apart.
- Bring one leg behind you and lunge down so your knee touches the floor.
- As you bring your knee back to the start position, bring the dumbbells up to perform a bicep curl.
- Bring your foot up to the start position so that you're standing upright.
- Lower the dumbbells back down and perform the exercise with the other leg.

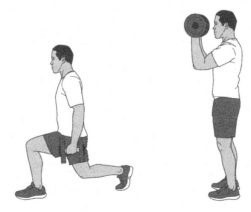

PUSH-UP TO SIDE PLANK TWIST

You're using your own bodyweight, so you're testing your strength while also engaging your core. The twisting movement means it's not so linear, and you're working in a different plane of movement.

- Get into the conventional push-up position. This can be performed with your hands on the floor or on a pair of light dumbbells or even a pair of push-up handles.
- As you get to the top of your push-up, take one hand off the floor and bring it behind your back.
- Twist around 45 degrees so you're focusing on that hand.
- Hold for a breath and then return to the start position.

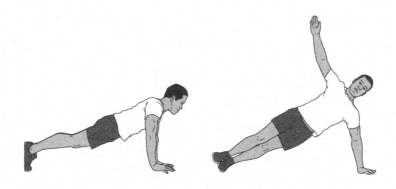

CLEANS TO SHOULDER PRESS WITH SQUAT THRUST AND BENT-OVER ROW

This is an exceptionally multifunctional exercise and is very cardiovascular. You need coordination, strength and agility. The combination of exercises is not for the faint-hearted, but once you have mastered them they are fast and efficient.

- Walk up to the bar with your feet shoulder-width apart and pick it up using an overhand grip.
- Keep a neutral neck and spine, drive the bar up, with your elbows high. As your elbows reach shoulder level, flip the bar over into a shoulder press position.
- Perform a shoulder press, pushing the weight above you into the air before bringing the bar back down to your chest and then to your thighs and then to the ground.
- Put your hands on the ground, shoot your legs out behind you and then shoot them back.
- Return to the original position, holding the bar, and perform a bent-over row.
- Lower the bar to your chest and down to your waist, and then return to the start position with neutral spine and neck.

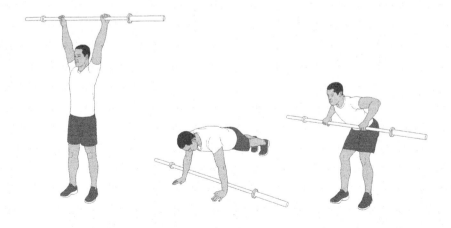

ADAM'S WORKOUT

Dead lift to squat thrust x 25 reps

Cardio

Dead lift to squat thrust x 20 reps

Squat thrust to pull-up x 20 reps

Cardio

Dead lift to squat thrust x 15 reps

Squat thrust to pull-up x 15 reps

Reverse lunge to bicep curl sequence x 15 reps on
each side

Cardio

Dead lift to squat thrust x 10 reps

Squat thrust to pull-up x 10 reps

Reverse lunge to bicep curl sequence x 10 reps on
each side

Push-up to side plank twist x 10 reps

Cardio

Dead lift to squat thrust x 8 reps

Squat thrust to pull-up x 8 reps

Reverse lunge to bicep curl sequence x 8 reps on
each side

Push-up to side plank twist x 8 reps

Cleans to shoulder press with squat thrust and
bent-over row x 8 reps

Cardio

8 | RELY ON YOURSELF, NOT MACHINES

Working out in a cave sounds bizarre. But I designed a gym inside one for Daniel Craig for *No Time to Die*, and we were perfectly happy to be in that space. That was when we were on location in Matera, an ancient city in southern Italy that is carved out of the hillside, and the most extraordinary place I've ever been to. The gym that I set up was very basic with just a few simple bits of kit. I didn't need anything complicated to train with Daniel, just somewhere clean and functional.

When I'm on location with actors, we might not have access to the same kit that we would normally use in our regular gym. The gym in the cave was quite unusual compared to the one at Pinewood Studios. When you're somewhere unfamiliar, you have to work and make adjustments according to what you have, but that can be a huge positive as it creates natural diversity and forces you to try new things. When I accompanied Daniel to Jamaica for his last Bond film, we embraced being in a different place with different kit. This goes to back to my old military days when we were taught to improvise, adapt and overcome.

While working on seven Bond films, I was fortunate enough to travel to some remarkable locations. One of the most memorable sites was the Cerro Paranal mountain in the Atacama Desert in Chile, which is more than 2,600 metres above sea level and one of the driest and most inhospitable places on Earth. It's usually only scientists who stay up there – as there's an observatory – and when Daniel was shooting scenes for *Quantum of Solace* we had to adapt to their gym facilities, as well as get used to training at high altitude.

DON'T GET ATTACHED TO STUFF

Sometimes on location, there might not be any kit at all. But I never use that as an excuse not to work out, and you shouldn't either. I like to be able to train anywhere. When I was prepping Benedict Cumberbatch for *Doctor Strange*, we would go to a park near his home in London and often make the most of the outdoor gym space. I would bring a bag with some kit in it to enable us to exercise outside, which was motivating and gave him a sense of freedom.

I'm always telling my clients not to become reliant on certain pieces of equipment as they don't have to be in their own gym, or indeed any gym, to maximize their results. Work with what you've got and what's always with you – your own body. Using your bodyweight and natural movement, you can create the intensity that you need, whether you're indoors or outdoors, at home or in the gym, at the park or on the track. You should have the self-confidence to train anywhere. From pull-ups, dips and lunges to squats and push-ups, you can utilize your bodyweight within a workout. When you've got access to more comprehensive bits of kit, fine, but know that when you don't have those machines, you can revert to your bodyweight exercises and still train effectively.

Instead of being reliant on machines, gizmos and gadgets, be reliant on yourself. All you need is your body and a workout theory or method that you can take anywhere with you. Invest in a theory and method before you invest in any kit or a gym membership.

ELIMINATE EXCUSES

Many of us look for excuses not to do something. Let's suppose you're on holiday or a business trip, and the hotel gym doesn't have the same equipment that you're used to at home; if you're dependent on certain machines, it's easy to use that as a reason not to work out or to do a shorter, less intense session.

When you're looking around a gym at the machines, you should remember that they're just inanimate things. You should always be thinking more about your body, and how you're going to move and create intensity. It's about shifting your mindset to how you view and interpret a workout space. You might spot a machine that's suitable for your upper body, but if you weren't in the gym, and you didn't have access to that piece of kit, you could do push-ups instead – you're still going to be training the same muscle groups.

Once you start giving more thought to your own body, you'll find that you become more creative regarding how you work out. Don't put restrictions on yourself when your imagination is endless. In the past, I've often had to adapt to my environment to carry out my job, whether it's getting actors to go up and down flights of stairs or to run in the sand in London's Hyde Park (which is meant for the horses). One of the benefits of being imaginative – and I write about this in the chapter about leaving your comfort zone – is that it forces you to do something you've never done before.

I always have a bag of bits ready to sling in the car and take anywhere with me. It contains some resistance bands, a TRX strap, an ab roller, some push-up handles, skipping ropes, pads and a mat. With those key items, I know I'll never be without a workout, wherever I go. Because of the hours that we work in the movie industry, you can never be sure the hotel gym will be open at the time you want to train. Or once at the gym, we might find that it's extremely busy. That's why that bag goes everywhere with me when I'm working on location. Why not have your own bag of kit packed? Then you'll always be ready for a workout. If an opportunity presents itself, you can use that time and energy to train.

DON'T WAIT FOR MACHINES

If someone is on a machine in the gym that you had planned to use next – and this will be a regular problem in busy gyms – don't just wait around until it's free: use the time to do something else. This is why it's so important to be aware of your body and the muscle groups that you want to train. By knowing your own body, you can switch to a different exercise that will work those muscles, and so you're not wasting time hanging about.

If you don't keep active your heart rate will start to drop, you'll begin to cool down and your motivation may start to ebb away. You'll also be wasting time. Instead, slide something else in there which is going to exercise the same muscle group. Remember, there are no rules. You should be glad to do something a bit different to get some diversity. If there are no machines available, use your own bodyweight to produce a similar movement. Just do something to keep your heart rate high and maintain the momentum and intensity of your workout. Try to keep moving from one exercise to the next.

USE NATURE AS YOUR GYM

You don't need to join a gym to get fit. Use nature as your gym – that could be parks or fields or your garden, as that's great for your stimulation and mental health.

Even if you're a member of a gym, try to mix it up and maybe use the gym in winter and go outside more in the summer. You don't want to tie yourself down to only doing one thing. You can do anything you want whenever you want. Use what's around you, keep things interesting and change your environment to suit your mood. I often think the best way to see any city, or anywhere new, is to go for a couple of runs. Or a walk. Get out and about, use your environment and get some mental stimulation from your workout.

When we were on location in Matera, Daniel and I enjoyed a spectacular walk through the old city to our gym cave, but we couldn't run as the cobblestones had been polished smooth by all the tourists – it would have been dangerous for us to move at speed on those slippery, steep streets and stairs, especially when it had been raining. But if we had been almost anywhere else, we would have been running and exploring simultaneously.

9 | DON'T LET AGE HOLD YOU BACK

Daniel Craig was in his late thirties when he played James Bond for the first time. By his final Bond film he was in his early fifties. But Daniel didn't ask less of himself because he was a little older. And I expected just as much from him, if not more.

From his first to his fifth appearance as 007, Daniel and I had maintained our high standards and showed what was possible within the movie industry. Some twenty-five-year-olds who work out a lot might like to think they're super fit and in amazing shape, but Daniel could probably hold his own alongside them. Nowadays, you don't have to be in your twenties or thirties to be an action hero. Who says that you can't look better at fifty than you did when you were in your twenties? The answer: no one at all. Daniel and I just thought, screw it, let's just go for it and see what we can do.

The fact that the movie industry no longer just wants young actors to play action roles is a reflection of the paradigm shift on fitness in society as a whole, I think. We've stopped seeing age as a barrier to good health, and I hope this continues. You can still have the same fitness goals as you did when you were younger, but you just have to take a different route, and probably more time, to get there. I needed around seven months to train Daniel for *Casino Royale*, but for his second Bond film, *Quantum of Solace*, the process took a little longer, lasting around nine months. Training Daniel for *Skyfall* took just under a year, and then I needed more time with him for *Spectre* and a bit longer again for *No Time to Die*.

You won't necessarily train and recover in your fifties exactly as you did in your thirties. We obviously can't completely ignore how our bodies change as we age, but we can also recognize that we're perhaps a little smarter, that we understand our bodies a little more and are more aware of what does and doesn't motivate us.

I like training actors who are a little older – it's very satisfying to ensure that they're completely prepared athletically when they turn up on set. When designing a programme for Harrison Ford for the fifth Indiana Jones film, for example, I had to consider the specific movement that would allow him to crack a whip, which is key for playing that character. While he was in his late seventies when he shot that movie, he wanted to do as much physical stuff as possible, and my programme gave him the flow and flexibility that he needed.

I've even had instances when the director and writers have adjusted the script to make the most of how incredibly fit their actor is at the start of filming. Sometimes the production team would remark: 'Oh my God, we didn't think he'd be able to do that, but let's utilize his athleticism and add a few new elements.' Perhaps the director had been planning on using a stuntman for a particular scene and then the actor turns up athletically capable. The director would ask the actor if he was willing and able to do the stunt himself, which is great for the film as it provides a much better and more authentic shot. Actors are normally happy to give it a go as that can be a fun part of the movie-making process.

GETTING MORE FROM YOUR WORKOUT

When you're younger, your metrics tend to be based on how much you're lifting, how fast you're running and how much you weigh. As you age, you can change how you measure your progress slightly, so it becomes more about how you're feeling and performing. When you're older, it becomes even more important for you to enjoy your workouts, and that training is making you happy. Do what makes you feel good – that's the most essential thing. With age, the balance changes. It used to be tipped towards being more athletic. But in your later years, it's more about maintaining health and wellbeing, and having lots of energy and flexibility.

Take Ralph Fiennes, for instance, who is exceptionally strong – far more so than you probably imagine. I've trained Ralph for his role as M in the Bond movies, for *Wrath of the Titans* and for various theatre productions. While Ralph is dedicated and interested in metrics – such as how much he can dead lift and bench-press – he has mentally adjusted them to be more age-appropriate (the metric for now should not be the metric you used when you were twenty-five). I feel as though, while he is training to be in great shape for movies, and he always told me he wanted to improve his posture and how he looked and moved in a suit, this also allows him to enjoy his life away from work (he is a total foodie).

LISTEN TO YOUR BODY

With age comes maturity and with maturity comes calculated decisions. You're listening to your body and giving it what it needs.

One of the great things about working with older actors, such as Harrison Ford, Woody Harrelson and Donnie Yen, is that it has often been an education for me. While I was teaching them, they were also teaching me, even though they might not have realized it. Someone like Woody has been in the industry for decades and has had so many professionals in his life who help him with his fitness and wellbeing. When I spoke to him during training programmes, I felt as though I was getting years of experience distilled into a few minutes of feedback. Woody challenged me, but I also gleaned some great snippets of information from him that I could then use with other clients. As a trainer, that kind of interaction can enhance your knowledge and help to make you unique in the industry.

Over the years, older actors have learned what they like and don't like. Take some time to listen to your own body and to understand what works for you. You're not going to recover at the age of fifty in the same way you did when you were twenty-one. That's just not physiologically possible. We don't create muscle tissue like we used to or move like we once did. The body isn't as efficient as it was back then. It's not producing the same standard of recovery aid or the same level of chemicals. Just as you have to train in an age-appropriate way, you have to recover in an age-appropriate way, too. Ideally, you should get used to doing lots of recovery when you're younger, so it becomes ingrained in your programme, and you'll carry on thinking it's a natural part of your lifestyle.

Donnie Yen is from the old school of doing his own stunts without padding. He's a respected martial artist. He's extremely fit, capable and proud. The big thing with Donnie, as I learned when helping him on *Rogue One: A Star Wars Story*, is his approach to recovery and how he makes sure he is helping his body to heal and repair. While Donnie still has an extreme level of fitness, he has adapted how he recovers as he knows that you can't keep doing the same things when you're older.

KEEP THINGS FRESH

Gerard Butler used to train in an old-school way – he was all about lifting and weight gain – and I tried to modernize his approach when preparing him for films, including on the thriller *London Has Fallen* and the submarine movie *Hunter Killer*. When I first started working with him, he wasn't training in an age-appropriate way – he was in his forties but was still trying to do things he had done in his twenties.

Some people are forever reflecting on what they did in the past rather than being in the present and focusing on what they can do now, as well as what they would like to do in the future. Gerard was a good example of this. He often talked about what he had done on old movies, such as *300* (mainly about the injuries he had incurred), but I told him that we would have to adapt his approach. I spoke to him about the importance of resetting his metrics and mindset to match his goals and age. You wouldn't want to work in the same way now that you did twenty years ago, but your results in the present can be just as good as those from the past – you just don't know it yet. It's important to feel as though you're working towards something fresh and new that's age-appropriate. You might have done something at a certain age to achieve a specific look, but we need to understand that as we get older, a new mental outlook and a new set of goals are needed.

Gerard listened to what I said and agreed to change his methods. The programme I designed for him didn't have rigid metrics that required him to lift a certain amount of weight, which had been the case in the past. As we age, it's important to have the mental capability to take a fresh approach and become a new, different version of yourself.

HARRISON FORD FOR
INDIANA JONES 5

Harrison is so **ENTHUSIASTIC** and so **INVESTED** in his
health. While he's in his late seventies, he's very
conscious of his overall wellbeing. He maintains a very
active, outdoorsy lifestyle, whether he's riding his
bike or his horse or playing tennis, which is one of his
passions. Harrison says that moving his body every
day keeps him **FRESH** and **HEALTHY**, and I think anyone –
no matter how old they are – should be inspired
by that.

With maturity comes **KNOWLEDGE**. Like Harrison, as
we get older, we begin to understand better what
our limitations are. You know what you're physically
capable of, but also what's not going to work.

As someone who has loved the Indiana Jones movies since childhood, it was a surreal moment when I found myself in a gym with Harrison Ford talking about the movements needed to crack a whip.

I remembered watching the original film, *Raiders of the Lost Ark*, as a young boy and it scared the hell out of me – particularly that terrifying scene towards the end, when the Ark of the Covenant was opened. All of the Indy films are iconic. And, forty years after *Raiders of the Lost Ark* was first shown in cinemas, I was hired to look after Harrison for the fifth Indiana Jones movie.

Harrison's a keen tennis player, so I think he was pleased to hear that the session I had designed for him would improve his serve, giving him a smoother action. It was almost as though cracking a whip was of secondary importance. I said to him: 'If you can serve a tennis ball, you'll be able to crack a whip like Indy. It's pretty much the same action.'

As background research, I watched some of the action scenes from past Indiana Jones films and, oh my God, he did some hardcore stuff back in the 1980s. That was a time when there wasn't much CGI (computer-generated imagery) to help you out, and he was performing most of his own stunts, raw and for real. Harrison was doing lots of running, jumping and hanging, with plenty of fight scenes and other choreography. For the leading man, the Indiana Jones movies can be as brutal to shoot as the Bond films – you're in almost every scene and everything revolves around you. You don't get any downtime. You're needed on set every day.

I thought it was commendable that, at his age, Harrison wanted to do another massive movie and was keen to do as much of the physical stuff as possible. He had a few niggles and injuries from all the action films he had done but, as long as he felt confident and capable, he was happy to do what he could. Harrison has always been fit. And look at how many action movies he has been in and the vast number of athletic scenes he has done.

Having been through the more challenging times in the 1980s, when he was essentially his own stuntman, for this Indiana Jones movie he was able to do things at his own pace rather than at anyone else's. He knew what he could manage and what he could leave for the stunt team to do.

The whips they use for Indiana Jones are quite heavy and there's a specific movement that Harrison had to do to crack them. It's like a snap. Of course, he had cracked the whip in four previous Indiana Jones films, but I designed a programme that would allow his body to move naturally and give him the flow and flexibility he would need for the new movie. It was also important that the programme gave him a feel-good factor and that he was pain-free. Harrison did this session twice a week while shooting the new Indiana Jones movie in 2021. I recommend this to readers of all ages, as it enables you to keep your body moving and your mind engaged. You're doing a session but you're being smart about it. It's smart because you're allowing the body to move naturally and without pain, but it still feels as though you're doing something – it's also going to help prevent soreness and pain. It's simply intelligent fitness.

ACTIVATION AND CARDIO

For activation, you can use resistance bands, bodyweight exercises, dynamic stretching or little bursts of controlled cardio. While I still adopted my go-to 5–2 method with Harrison, I swapped the usual two minutes of cardio between exercises for two minutes of using a percussion tool (a vibrating massage gun) on muscle tissue. I think it felt a little more like a recovery session for Harrison, rather than a full-on workout. If you want to do two minutes of cardio, feel free to jump on the bike or do whatever will raise your heart rate.

HARRISON'S 5-2 WORKOUT

SINGLE ARM LATERAL PULLDOWN WITH A BAND

Everything in Harrison's *Indiana Jones* workout involved bands rather than weights, as it provides a smoother action and a constant tension through the action. I would set up the bands on a rack or cage using a high band, a medium band around waist height and a low band, which are all good for stretching and distraction (when the blood flows between the joints). This particular exercise is good for your back and shoulders.

- While on your knees facing the cage, grab a high band that's connected to the top of the cage above your head. Grip the band with three fingers – not using the thumb or the little finger. This gives you better grip and feeling.
- Staying on your knees, gently shuffle back until the band is under tension.
- Keeping your elbow close to your body, pull the band down until it's level with your chest.

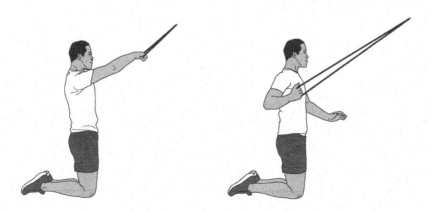

- Very slowly, and with controlled movement, let the band return to the cage. You're allowing the band to pull you slightly forward and it will feel as though the shoulder is being pulled gently out of its socket, but it's not. And this is allowing blood to flow between the joints.
- Now do the same with the other arm.

LATERAL ROTATION WITH A BAND

This exercise is good for your rotator cuff and for the rear postural muscles, and helps to prevent your shoulders from rolling forward.

- Stand to the side of the cage and grab the band that's at medium height, again using your first three fingers.
- Keep your elbow in tight to your side and rotate your arm away from you, until you feel some tension in the band.
- In a slow and controlled fashion, allow the band to return to the start position.
- Swap over and repeat on the other side.

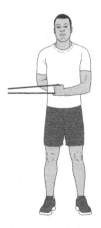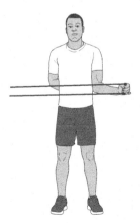

MEDIAL ROTATION WITH A BAND

You're exercising the same muscles here as in the previous lateral rotation exercise.

- Spin around 180 degrees, using the band that's at medium height, again gripping it using just three fingers.
- This time bring the band and the tension into your tummy button.
- Keep your core tight while you perform this exercise as this gives you the secondary benefit of the body having to stabilize itself.
- Swap over and repeat on the other side.

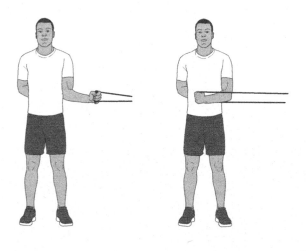

SINGLE ARM LOW ROW WITH A BAND

This exercise trains your rear delts and lats.

- Using the low band, again use three fingers to grip it with one hand.
- While keeping your elbow close to your body, pull the band towards you until your hand reaches the side of your chest. That will allow you to squeeze the lat, which is the side of your back.
- Now release and let the band go back to its original position.
- Swap over and do the other arm.

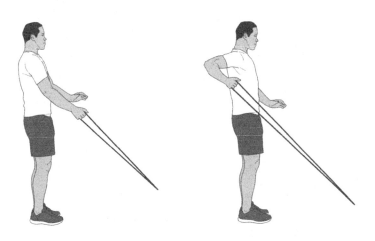

SHOULDER CAPSULE STRETCH WITH A BAND

In addition to your shoulders, this exercise also trains your chest, biceps and forearms.

- Face away from the cage, with a high band dangling down behind you.
- Grab the band with both hands, using the first three fingers on each hand to hold it.
- Walk away until there is tension in the band, with your head down so your arms are slightly raised behind you.
- Gradually step forward with one foot and raise your head until you are focusing forward and then gently start to elevate your chest. You will feel the shoulder capsule (the soft and connective tissues) stretch.
- Maintain that stretch for 30–60 seconds.
- Gently walk backwards towards the cage and release your fingers as you return to the start position.

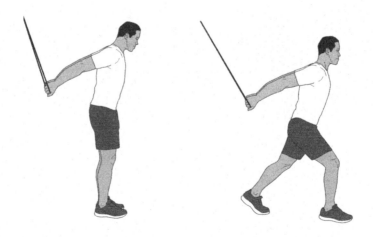

HARRISON'S WORKOUT

Single arm lateral pulldown with a band x 15 reps
   on each side

Percussion tool: lats

Single arm lateral pulldown with a band x 12 reps
   on each side
Lateral rotation with a band x 12 reps on each side

Percussion tool: shoulders

Single arm lateral pulldown with a band x 10 reps
   on each side
Lateral rotation with a band x 10 reps on each side
Medial rotation with a band x 10 reps on each side

Percussion tool: shoulders

Single arm lateral pulldown with a band x 8 reps
   on each side
Lateral rotation with a band x 8 reps on each side
Medial rotation with a band x 8 reps on each side
Single arm low row with a band x 8 reps on each side

Percussion tool: low back and lats

Single arm lateral pulldown with a band x 6 reps
   on each side
Lateral rotation with a band x 6 reps on each side
Medial rotation with a band x 6 reps on each side
Single arm low row with a band x 6 reps on each side
Shoulder capsule stretch with a band: stretch for 30–60
   seconds

Percussion tool: shoulder capsule

JOHN KRASINSKI FOR
JACK RYAN

H

I completely respect the way John goes about his business. In almost every session, I found myself saying to him, 'Don't do too much, **DON'T OVERLOAD** the bar, you don't need to prove a point to yourself today,' and occasionally I had to rein him in. I never had to say, 'You're not doing enough.'

John has **PURE NATURAL STRENGTH**, as well as drive and ambition, and like any actor he is **METICULOUS** with his preparations for a film. Watching someone work that hard – especially someone who has a busy life, as a husband and a father – is always **INSPIRATIONAL**.

John says he always likes to be within three to four weeks of his best body. He understands it's physically impossible to be at the highest standard of fitness all the time. It would be crazy to imagine you can be forever at your optimum as it's simply not realistic nor sustainable.

In that way, John thinks like an elite athlete, which is the mindset that actors need in today's action-movie business. Every athlete will tell you that you try to peak for certain events, such as the Olympics, but that you can only maintain that level for a few weeks and then you have to drop down from such heights for a less intense period. After you've rested your body and mind, you can start resetting your goals and begin building up to your best once again.

Before training John, I worked with his wife, Emily Blunt, while preparing her for *The Adjustment Bureau*. John and Emily don't just work out for films; it's become part of their natural lifestyle to have good health and wellbeing. But when they want to get themselves ready for a role, they can adjust their focus and ramp it up a bit. When they're changing their performance and aesthetic for a part, it is helpful to have a strong foundation from which to start. They're always able to push the button when the need arises, and that's essential for mind and body. And then when a project is over, they can bring it down, but fitness is still going to be key to their lifestyle.

John was playing Jack Ryan, a CIA agent, so he wanted to look as though he could handle himself in the field. He had to be able to do multiple athletic things – sprint, fight, bounce off a wall, and take a gun apart and put it back together again. The role demanded speed and hand–eye coordination.

To prepare John for a long shoot, I designed a thorough, intense programme, which included a sprinkling of what John likes. And what John liked was big strength capability. His favourite barometer was the one-rep max (as much weight as you can lift with one repetition), as it's easy to be competitive with your training partner or buddy.

This workout is an example of what John endured when he was in the muscle-building phase of trying to reach his peak. These are big, big exercises. After the build-up phase, we would switch to more of a conditioning phase to help reveal all of that well-earned muscle tissue.

If you want to remain within a few weeks of your best body at all times, you need to know how to train and maintain in a sustainable way that lets you reach your optimum and also allows you to stay there for a while. It's important that when you're in your sustaining mode, you still feel as though you have somewhere to go and more to give. If you leave yourself with nothing in your toolbox when you're ready to take it to your peak, that will make things very difficult.

If you use strength as your metric, frequently go back to the key, original compound exercises and see where your one-rep max is. John and I would do this once every four to six weeks to check if he was stronger or maintaining his strength from the last measurement. It's easier to monitor your progression with a one-rep max as you don't pre-fatigue the muscle. Even when you're not at your optimum, you should be able to maintain your strength to ensure you keep within 20 per cent of your one-rep max.

ACTIVATION AND CARDIO

For activation, John would tackle an incline on the treadmill for ten minutes. As he walked, I'd talk through what was on the whiteboard in the gym, with the preparations very intense for that role. John did a mix of cardio for this workout, including two minutes of sprinting on the treadmill for the first lot, riding on the assault bike for the second (which involves using handles as well as pedalling), and going on the Versaclimber machine that simulates climbing for the third. He sprinted on the treadmill for the fourth lot of cardio, and for the fifth burst he was back on the assault bike again.

JOHN'S 5–2 WORKOUT

HEAVY BENCH PRESS

It's not how fast the bar is moved up and down, but the time that the muscle is under tension or contraction that will give you the most adaptation and allow you to make the biggest gains. You can mix things up with this exercise, including using different angles on the bench, from incline to flat to decline.

- You'll need a training buddy to act as your spotter (or ask someone in the gym to help you). Alternatively, you can use a Smith machine to hook a bar on and off for safety.
- Lie back on a flat bench. The foot position is entirely down to you depending on what you find most comfortable. Some people like to have their feet on the bench, while others prefer to put their feet on the floor, on either side of the bench.
- Take the bar with your hands positioned just over shoulder-width apart.
- You should be helped with the first part of the exercise, especially when there's a lot of weight on the bar.
- Slowly lower the bar to your chest.
- Explode back to the start position with your elbows locked out or straight.

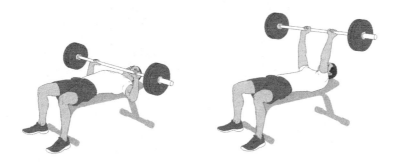

HEAVY DEAD LIFT

Compound exercises were the cornerstone of John's workout as they meant he was always recruiting multiple muscle groups, and this allowed him not only to have muscle growth but also strength gains.

- Stand in front of a barbell with your feet shoulder-width apart and your toes pointing forward. Focus directly ahead of you.
- Arrange one hand with an overhand grip and one with an underhand grip.
- With a neutral back and neck, bend down and pick up the bar, and then return to the standing position, with the bar gently touching the middle of your thighs. You should be leaning back very slightly.
- Take the bar back to mid-shin or the floor, depending on your ability and range of movement.

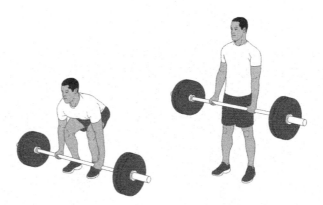

HEAVY SQUATS

I love squats. I can't think of a muscle group that you don't make use of while squatting, so this is also going to put pressure on your cardiovascular system. Squats are the most fluid muscle sequence that the body can perform. The gains are immense and the benefits are noticeable. If you wish, you can do this exercise with dumbbells rather than a bar.

- Try to use a neck pad as that adds some comfort.
- Stand in front of the weights bar, which should be around shoulder height.
- With your feet positioned shoulder-width apart, lift the bar off carefully, hold in position at shoulder height and take two steps back while still focusing forward.
- Point your toes slightly outwards.
- Squat down, sticking your bottom out, until your knees are at 90 degrees.
- Pause and return to the start position.

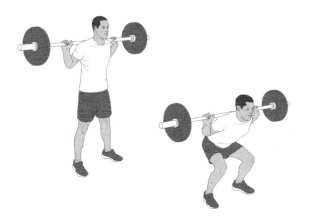

PULL-UPS

What could be better than using your own bodyweight and lifting yourself over a bar? If you lose a few kilos of body fat, and gain a little bit more strength, you'll find that the pull-up is a lot easier. A pull-up is a very visual, motivational exercise.

- Using an overhand grip, put your hands on the pull-up bar just over shoulder-width apart.
- Cross your ankles and raise your heels until they are at a 90-degree angle – this will stop you from rocking around and ensure you engage the right muscles.
- Pull yourself up until your chin is slightly above the bar. Return to the start position.
- If you struggle with this exercise, add a resistance band under your feet which will act as a counterbalance, so you're no longer lifting all of your bodyweight. Alternatively, you could put a bench or a chair beneath the pull-up bar, which will enable you to jump up before you slowly lower yourself down.

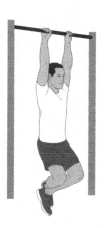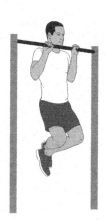

DIPS

Similar to pull-ups, dips give you the great feeling of using your own bodyweight to get stronger, and again it's a great metric of your progression. Being able to lower yourself down and then return back to a start position is a very satisfying feeling.

- Put your hands on the edge of something stable, such as a bench. Your hands are behind you and shoulder-width apart. Your legs are raised, preferably above waist height.
- Lower yourself down so your elbows are at 90 degrees.
- Now push back to the start position.
- Remember to exhale on exertion.

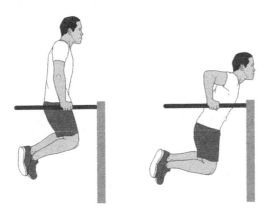

JOHN'S WORKOUT

Heavy bench press x 25 reps

Cardio

Heavy bench press x 20 reps
Heavy dead lift x 20 reps

Cardio

Heavy bench press x 15 reps
Heavy dead lift x 15 reps
Heavy squats x 15 reps

Cardio

Heavy bench press x 10 reps
Heavy dead lift x 10 reps
Heavy squats x 10 reps
Pull-ups x 10 reps

Cardio

Heavy bench press x 8 reps
Heavy dead lift x 8 reps
Heavy squats x 8 reps
Pull-ups x 8 reps
Dips x 8 reps

Cardio

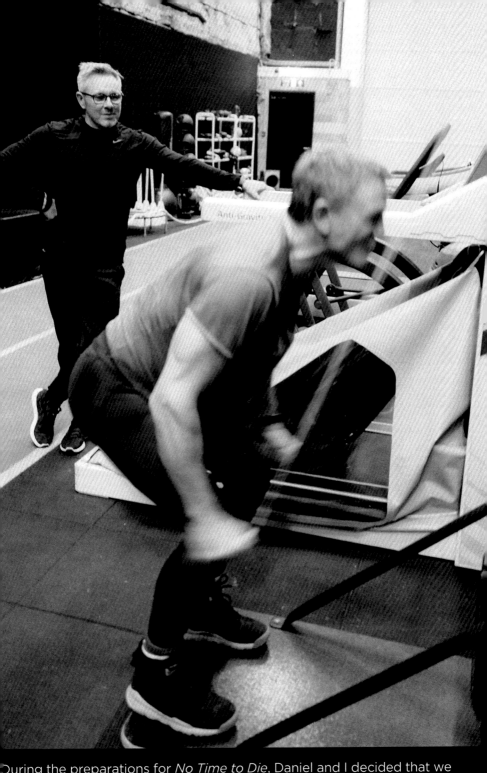

During the preparations for *No Time to Die*, Daniel and I decided that we

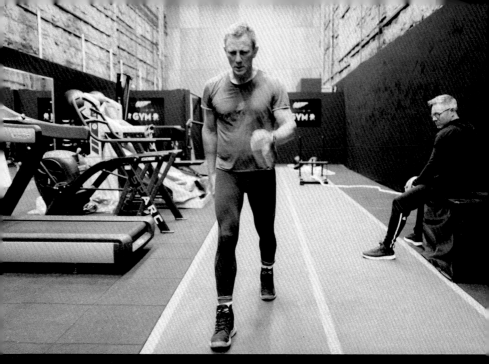

ABOVE. Keeping a strong mentality is just as important as a strong physicality.

BELOW. Even when Daniel had an injury setback and his lower body wasn't functioning, his upper body was still capable and we always kept training.

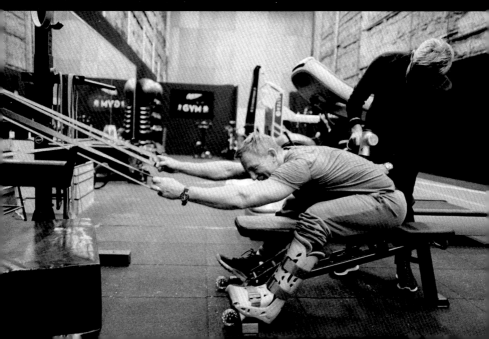

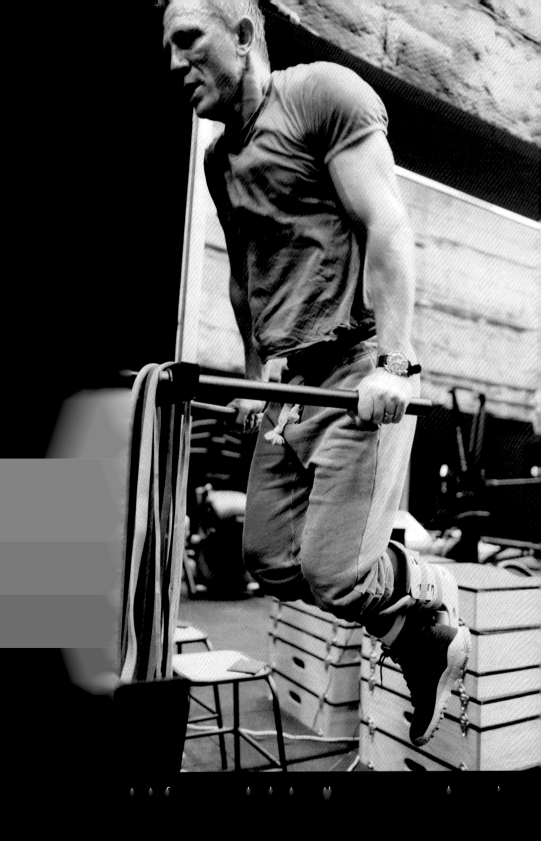

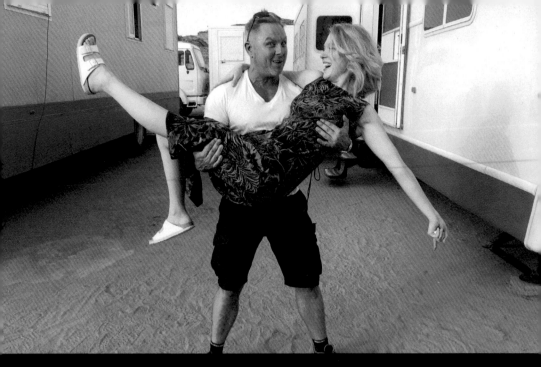

ABOVE. On location with Léa Seydoux in Morocco while shooting *Spectre*. Léa was extremely dedicated to the workouts I created to prepare her for *Spectre* and *No Time to Die*.

BELOW LEFT. Benedict Cumberbatch prepares for *Dr Strange 2*.

BELOW RIGHT. I've always found it more rewarding helping others achieve their fitness goals than working towards my own, but I've got to keep up!

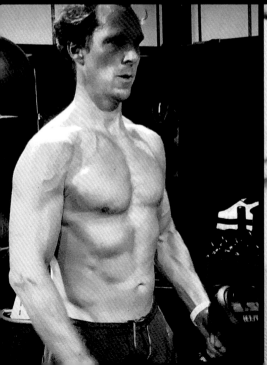

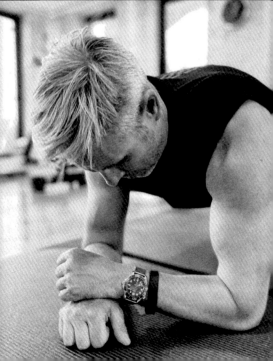

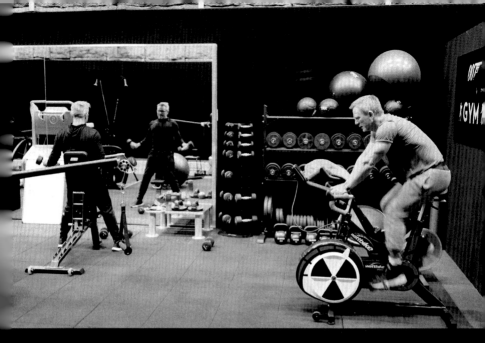

ABOVE. Daniel and I inside the Bond gym at Pinewood – with the 007 branding on the wall serving as a reminder of why he was working so hard.

BELOW. Daniel cracking on with the rehab for *No Time to Die* – the work didn't stop just because his foot was injured.

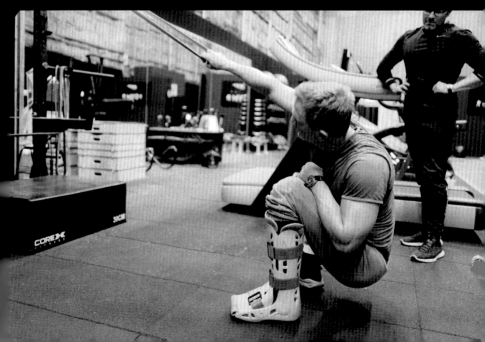

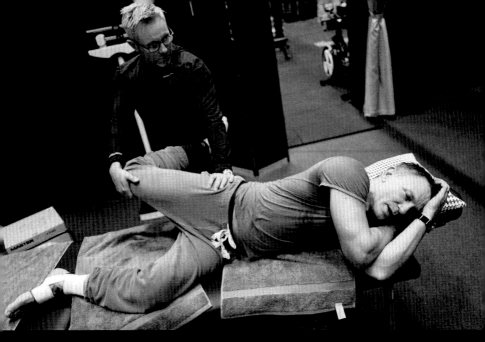

ABOVE. Stretching Daniel on *No Time to Die* – it was really important to keep o top of his recovery during filming.

BELOW. Stretching was an integral part of Daniel's programme for every Bond movie.

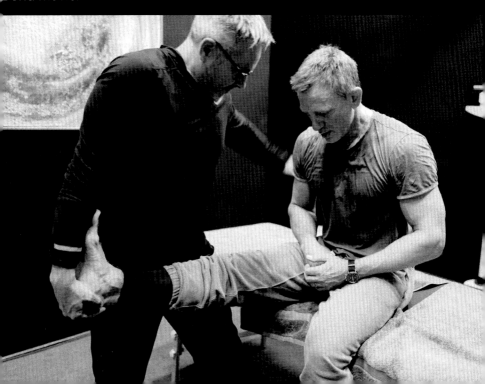

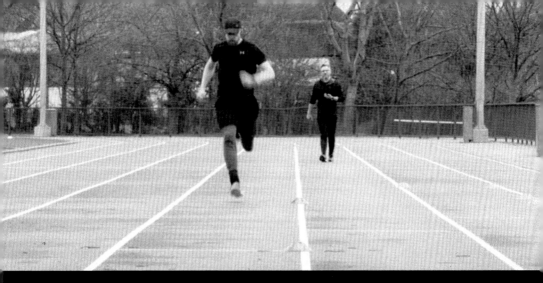

ABOVE. Tom Hiddleston doing sprint drills at his local track in London while preparing for *Kong: Skull Island*.

BELOW. Tom stretching after completing his drills.

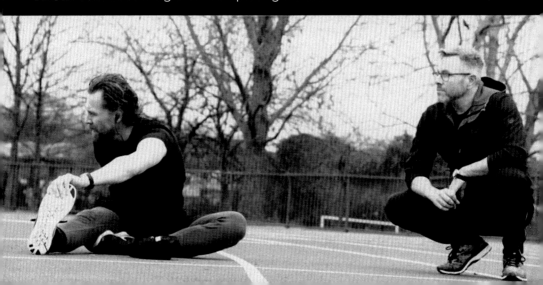

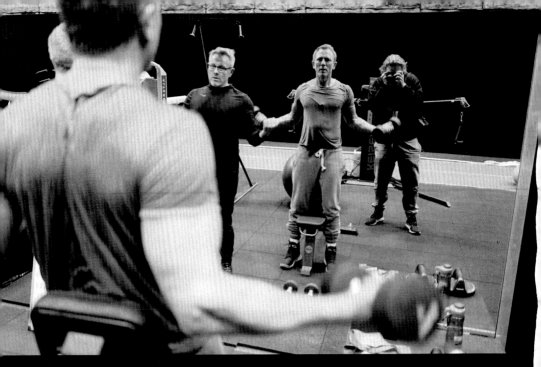

ABOVE. All in it together. Me, Daniel and official Bond photographer Greg Williams inside the *No Time to Die* gym.

BELOW. In a role reversal, here I am being trained by Bond. Daniel took this picture of the two of us a few weeks before the premiere for *No Time to Die* in August 2021.

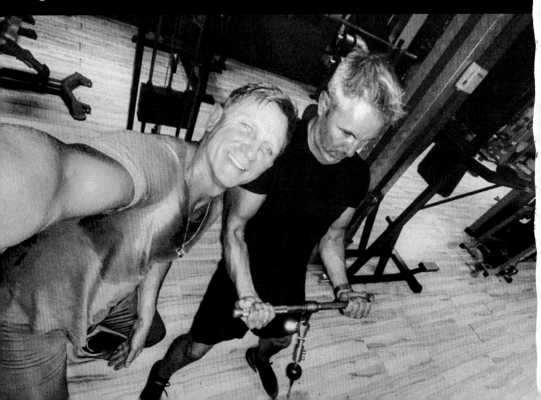

BENEDICT CUMBERBATCH FOR
DOCTOR STRANGE

H

Benedict is very **CHARACTER-DRIVEN** – he changes his physicality for every role to ensure it matches up with the personality and presence. From movie to movie, he is always adapting his workouts and **TRYING NEW THINGS**. For instance, while he was bigger for a role like *Doctor Strange*, he would have had to have lost some weight for a film such as *The Imitation Game*. Benedict has the **NATURAL DIVERSITY** that everyone should be looking for in life. We should all be trying new things.

Benedict is a busy person, but he was always there, however early or late it was, to put in the work. **TIME AND EFFICIENCY** were always key with him. I adapted his workouts to suit his heavy work schedule, which is what I believe we all need to do.

Doctor Strange was Benedict Cumberbatch's first Marvel movie, which is a big moment in anyone's career. Stepping into the Marvel Cinematic Universe is daunting as you know there will be certain demands and expectations. You're aware there's going to be a lot of athleticism and movement, as well as plenty of action sequences, which are difficult at the best of times and even more challenging when wearing a restrictive costume.

I knew from day one that Benedict would handle his first Marvel production with precision and ease, as he was exceptionally capable and invested. I wasn't getting a complete novice – he had trained before. I had three or four months to give Benedict the tools he needed to move, look and feel like his character, and do whatever he was asked on set. Benedict was meticulous but, most of all, he trusted in my process and was willing to do what it took to ensure he had the right conditioning and aesthetic for that movie.

While one of our goals was moulding Benedict's physique and giving him a little more functional muscle mass that he needed for the shoot, I was aware that it couldn't look contrived, as if his body was developed from going to the gym and working out. The director wanted Benedict's physique to appear as though it was a product of the character's lifestyle. We followed a very similar training programme for the sequel, *Dr Strange 2*.

ACTIVATION AND CARDIO

Benedict's a super-quick 100-metre sprinter, and so I would design sprint drills on a track for the cardio portion of his workout and gradually increase their intensity. I would start by asking him to do the first 100-metre sprint at 40 per cent of his maximum capability, then for the second one he would be running at 60 per cent, the third at 80 per cent and lastly he would do a couple at full intensity. Occasionally we would leave the track and do some hill sprints instead. At the end of this workout, we would normally run back to his house and then cool down, stretch and hydrate.

BENEDICT'S 5–2 WORKOUT

PARALLEL BAR DIPS

I liked to use the parallel bars because there was an amazing bit of kit that was available in the park. The great thing about parallel bars is that they offer a full bodyweight exercise, so they're ideal for development, strength and allowing you to push your capabilities.

- Getting yourself onto the parallel bars is normally the hardest part. With your elbows locked out or straight, your legs in a 90-degree position and your ankles crossed at the back, lower yourself until your elbows are at 90 degrees.
- Return to the start position, locking out or straightening your elbows.
- Always do as many as you can in a controlled way without rocking. As you start to tire, help yourself by putting your feet or ankles on a resistance band so you can squeeze out the last few reps (you might find it easier to put the band there before you start the exercise).

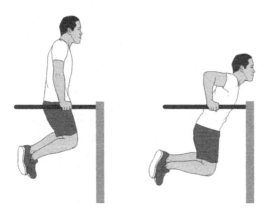

PARALLEL BAR PUSH-UPS

Using your bodyweight is a great barometer of your progression. It's simplistic and easy to control. It's also very safe as you're not doing movements with a high risk of injury.

- You can do these on parallel bars or on any other push-up handles or even dumbbells. Having your wrists in a straighter position allows you to go deeper into the push-up, adding more resistance and movement.
- Always ensure you have a neutral neck or back, with your core engaged and your tailbone tucked under. Your feet should be shoulder-width apart.
- Lower yourself until your chest is slightly below the bars and then return to the start position with your elbows locked.

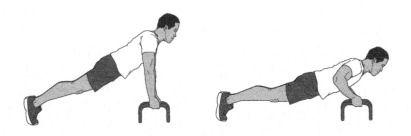

PULL-UPS

Doing pull-ups is another great barometer of your strength. Any activity involving your own bodyweight can be challenging and helps to build mass.

- Using an overhand grip, put your hands on the pull-up bar just over shoulder-width apart.
- Cross your ankles and raise your heels until they are at a 90-degree angle – this will stop you from rocking around and ensure you engage the right muscles.
- Pull yourself up until your chin is slightly above the bar. Return to the start position.
- If you struggle with this exercise, add a resistance band under your feet which will act as a counterbalance, so you're no longer taking all of your bodyweight. Alternatively, you could put a bench or a chair beneath the pull-up bar, which enables you to jump up before you slowly let yourself down.

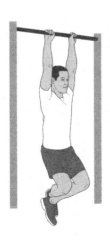 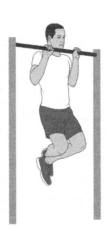

TRICEP DIPS WITH LEGS RAISED

As well as being great for triceps, this exercise is good for stretching out the capsules of your shoulders, which are the ligaments around the joints. It's also easy to adapt, as you could do it with one leg. I would increase resistance with Benedict by putting him in a weighted vest. Another way of building up intensity when you're on the upward portion of the exercise is to look slightly up in the air and then almost behind you.

- Put your hands on the edge of something stable, such as a bench. Your hands are behind you shoulder-width apart. Your feet and ankles should be resting on a bench in front of you, preferably above waist height.
- Lower yourself down so your elbows are at 90 degrees.
- Now push back to the start position.
- Remember to exhale on exertion.

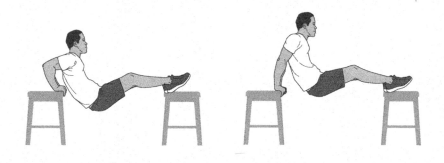

TRX BICEPS

The TRX is a versatile piece of kit that allows you to adjust your resistance by moving your body position to engage more or less bodyweight. This exercise is a great finisher to any workout as it allows you to use up the last 10 per cent of your body's capacity and reach failure, which means you can no longer complete another rep, using a very natural movement.

- Adopting an underhand grip and taking a moderate amount of your bodyweight, bring the palms of your hands to your forehead.
- Squeeze the bicep and return to the original position with your elbows locked out or straight.
- If you require more resistance, move your feet forward and lean further back. If you favour less resistance, bring your feet back towards you so you're almost in a standing position.

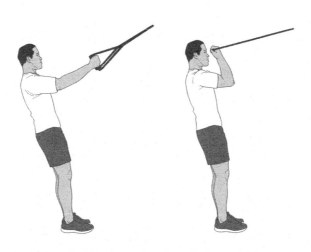

BENEDICT'S WORKOUT

Parallel bar dips x 25 reps

Cardio

Parallel bar dips x 20 reps
Parallel bar push-ups x 20 reps

Cardio

Parallel bar dips x 15 reps
Parallel bar push-ups x 15 reps
Pull-ups x 15 reps

Cardio

Parallel bar dips x 10 reps
Parallel bar push-ups x 10 reps
Pull-ups x 10 reps
Tricep dips with legs raised x 10 reps

Cardio

Parallel bar dips x 8 reps
Parallel bar push-ups x 8 reps
Pull-ups x 8 reps
Tricep dips with legs raised x 8 reps
TRX biceps x 8 reps

Cardio

TOM HIDDLESTON FOR
KONG: SKULL ISLAND

H

Tom's **COMPETITIVE**. But he's competitive with himself as well as with other people, and that's a great attribute to have. He would measure himself based on how many pull-ups he could do and what his one-rep max was for exercises, and also test how fast he could run 5 kilometres. **DON'T BE AFRAID** of setting yourself some challenges.

Preparing for *Kong* was a huge, huge challenge. But Tom loved it – he was **HAPPY TO GIVE ANYTHING AND EVERYTHING A GO**. He was often out of his comfort zone, but he was perfectly OK doing things he normally wouldn't. I think everyone can be inspired by the mentality that Tom brought to getting in shape for that movie.

Tom welcomed the intensity and the pain. For him, it seemed to be the more pain the better. He didn't mind being on the edge of throwing up in every session (though, of course, I wouldn't recommend this approach!).

When I created a programme for Tom to get him ready for *Kong: Skull Island*, a modern take on King Kong, he said to me: 'I'm happy to be out of my comfort zone as long as that gets me to where I need to be.' With that mentality, I knew that Tom would be able to handle anything I asked him to do in the gym. He really could take the intensity. Of all the programmes I have created in more than twenty years in the movie industry, Tom's might have been the most brutal.

But it had to be tough if he was going to put on as much muscle tissue as genetically possible. We were using heavy compound exercises and we were hitting them hard. I needed him to do the exercises until failure, and then go into forced reps, which is when your training partner steps in to help you do a couple more reps after failure by taking some of the weight. But Tom was always glad to be doing it; he was willing to load up the bar with weights and endure the intensity if he felt that would help him to portray the character in the movie.

When you're training Tom, you really have to know what you're talking about as he is incredibly knowledgeable as well as being fit and strong. Before I started with him on *Kong*, he was already working out at a very high level, thanks to his genetics and also because he's been very active since he was young. As a boy, he played all sports and was a superb athlete. He was insanely talented when he was younger. Tom was a great rugby player and an amazing cross-country runner, and so that sporting background has helped him to be athletic in action movies.

While Tom was preparing for *Kong*, he was also working on the TV drama *The Night Manager*, as it's common for busy actors to be involved in filming for one production while getting ready to transition into the next. Under such circumstances, I have to be conscious of not changing someone's aesthetic too much as that could affect continuity on the original show. To help him build more muscles we changed his nutrition around, adding more calories with an emphasis on protein.

Another adjustment I had to make with Tom was to reduce the amount of time he spent running. For Tom, it's a form of escapism as he finds it relatively easy. He would sometimes run 10 kilometres in the morning for fun, but I had to limit that as I didn't want him going catabolic and burning through muscle tissue as energy. That's why it was imperative that his nutrition was just right. Otherwise, much of that hard work cultivating muscle tissue would have been wasted. Though I still encouraged Tom to go running, because that was what he loved, I asked him to compress it and to go out for shorter but more intense runs.

I chose the first four exercises in this workout – heavy dumbbell incline press, heavy dumbbell squats, heavy seated shoulder press and heavy dead lift – because they're massive compound exercises and I believe they are an efficient way of building muscle.

I wrote Tom's statistics on the whiteboard in the gym so that I always knew his maximum weight and his rep capability as we progressed through the weeks. For me, the metrics for Tom on that movie were how much he was lifting, how many calories he was consuming and how much muscle tissue he was gaining.

ACTIVATION AND CARDIO

Tom would quite often say to me, 'Let yourself into my place as I'm just going to do a quick 5-kilometre run.' That suited me as I would set everything up ready for his return. Thank God I didn't have to do the run with him as I would never have kept up. If you're not a keen runner, you can instead activate and fire up muscle tissue by using resistance bands or doing ballistic squats. If something feels good and helps to prepare you for the task in hand, you should always do it.

TOM'S 5–2 WORKOUT

HEAVY DUMBBELL INCLINE PRESS

This exercise gives you fantastic strength as well as shape. The angle of the bench – incline, flat, decline – determines where the emphasis of the exercise is, and where the firing of the muscle group starts. With an incline, you're working out a lot more of your upper chest as well as recruiting your shoulders a bit more.

- Vary the angle of the bench from session to session to change the emphasis of the muscle groups you're recruiting. Anything from 25 to 45 degrees is great.
- Lift the dumbbells off the floor onto your knees and then use some momentum to get them into the air and into position.
- Lift the dumbbells above your chest until they're gently touching.
- Bring the dumbbells down until your arms are at 90 degrees and you can feel a nice stretch across your chest.
- Return the dumbbells to the start position above the chest and lock out or straighten your elbows.
- Now lift the dumbbells up until they're kissing.

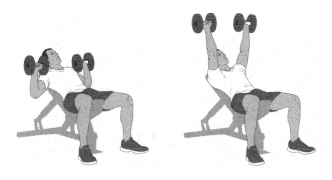

HEAVY DUMBBELL SQUATS

I see this as the jewel in the crown of all exercises as this is basically an all-over body workout in one. From the moment you pick up the weight to start the squat, your body is using almost every muscle group to create the power and the force to help you perform the exercise. The energy needed to execute a squat is immense.

- Stand with your feet shoulder-width apart with your toes pointing slightly away from you and the dumbbells on the floor on either side of your feet.
- Keeping a neutral back and neck, bend down and pick the dumbbells up.
- Engage the core and squeeze through the glutes and hamstrings. Gently lock out or straighten your knees and do a slight tilt of your pelvis to mark the end of a rep.
- Return to the start position. I like the dumbbells to touch the floor, but if your legs go to 90 degrees that's fine as well.

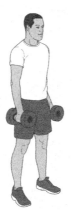 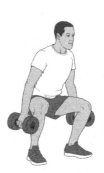

HEAVY SEATED SHOULDER PRESS

As well as being a big compound exercise and a great way of measuring your progression, a heavy seated shoulder press is also something you can play around with. How you position yourself is very important, as you can recruit secondary stabilizing muscles such as your core. You can also play around with hand positions, doing it with your palms facing you, which is known as an Arnold press (named after Arnold Schwarzenegger), as well as the more common shoulder press, when your palms face away from you.

- While seated on a bench, pick the dumbbells off the floor, lift them up and put them on your knees.
- Preferably have a training buddy or 'spotter' behind you as you use a little bit of momentum to get the dumbbells up into the shoulder-press position.
- Your buddy or spotter should help you to do the first rep into the air, with the dumbbells directly above your head. The dumbbells should gently kiss.
- Bring the dumbbells down until your elbows are at 90 degrees.
- Always make sure, as with any exercise, that you're breathing out with exertion. That's going to increase your power and strength.

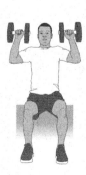
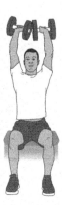

HEAVY DEAD LIFT

There are multiple formats for this exercise, and it's a great one for strength – including grip strength – and overall muscular development. You can choose whether you do this using dumbbells or barbells. You could try a variety of start positions: pick the bar up off the ground, or start from halfway down the shin or from just below the knee. You can also add another element, such as a plyometric and a press-up, while still holding the bar.

- Stand in front of a barbell with your feet shoulder-width apart and your toes pointing forward. Focus on looking directly ahead of you.
- I prefer to have one hand with an overhand grip and one with an underhand grip because I think that gives you more power and control.
- With a neutral back and neck, bend down and pick up the bar and return to the standing position, with the bar gently touching the middle of your thighs. You should be leaning back very slightly.
- Take the bar back to mid-shin or the floor, depending on your ability and range of movement.

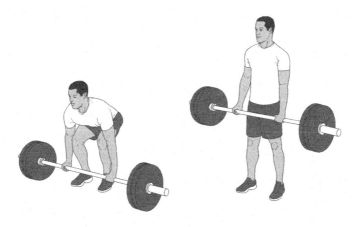

MATRIX OF FINISHERS

I liked to finish off the workout with a few exercises – tricep dips, push-ups and lateral raises – that ensure complete fatigue and failure in certain muscle groups. Don't be afraid of failure on these exercises as that's only going to help you achieve adaptation.

TRICEP DIPS

- Put your hands on the edge of something stable, such as a bench. Your hands are behind you and shoulder-width apart. Your legs and ankles are raised on a bench, preferably above waist height.
- Lower yourself down so your elbows are at 90 degrees.
- Now push back to the start position.
- Remember to exhale on exertion.

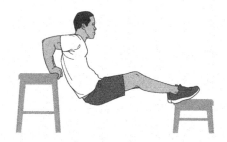

PUSH-UPS

- Put your hands on the floor shoulder-width apart.
- If you're new to this or you're at a lower level of ability, start on the top parts of your knees and have your legs crossed behind you.
- If you feel more comfortable, and to protect your wrists a bit more, you can hold two dumbbells, which will straighten your wrists and allow you to go further down.
- Lower yourself down until your elbows are at 90 degrees or go lower if you're using two dumbbells.

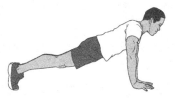

- Push up and return to the start position. Breathe out on exertion.
- To increase intensity, take your knees off the ground, keep a neutral back and neck, and do the same movement.

LATERAL RAISES

- Raise the dumbbells to the side with slightly bent elbows so they are parallel with your ears or the tops of your shoulders.
- Return to the start position.

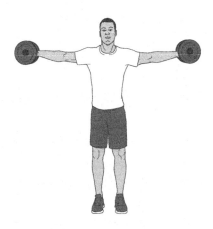

TOM'S WORKOUT

Heavy dumbbell incline press x 25 reps

Cardio

Heavy dumbbell incline press x 20 reps
Heavy dumbbell squats x 20 reps

Cardio

Heavy dumbbell incline press x 15 reps
Heavy dumbbell squats x 15 reps
Heavy seated shoulder press x 15 reps

Cardio

Heavy dumbbell incline press x 10 reps
Heavy dumbbell squats x 10 reps
Heavy seated shoulder press x 10 reps
Heavy dead lift x 10 reps

Cardio

Heavy dumbbell incline press x 8 reps
Heavy dumbbell squats x 8 reps
Heavy seated shoulder press x 8 reps
Heavy dead lift x 8 reps
Matrix of finishers x 8 reps

Cardio

BRYCE DALLAS HOWARD FOR
JURASSIC WORLD

You don't have to use strength or speed as your metric; Bryce's biggest goal was improving her **STABILITY** and **BALANCE**. When I started with her, she found it very difficult to stand on one leg on the ground. But after I had trained her for *Jurassic World*, she could easily stand on one leg unsupported on the BOSU ball, even with her eyes shut. Bryce was thrilled – that was **SUCH A BIG PROGRESSION** for her.

Bryce was always smiling and laughing, whether it was the beginning of the workout or the end. She was forever telling me how much she enjoyed some of the exercises, and I think that **POSITIVITY** helped her to get the most out of her workouts.

It felt as though Bryce spent months running around in high heels and a white trouser suit being chased by dinosaurs. You don't step into that scenario without first conditioning and preparing yourself.

When you're shooting an action movie like *Jurassic World*, it's said that you get about a minute of usable footage a day. As an actor, you're putting in twelve- or fourteen-hour days of running through the jungle, jumping on and off trucks and diving underneath cars, as well as sporadically fighting off a T-Rex. Some days, you won't even get those sixty seconds for all your efforts.

The periods of pre-production and shooting *Jurassic World* were extremely athletically demanding for Bryce. They are seriously long, brutal shoots, lasting around six months, and she could be on set from 6 a.m. until 6 p.m. each day. With schedules like this, you really need to know how to look after yourself, otherwise you're not going to get through it. My main aim is to limit and manage any niggles or injuries my actors may have, and try to prevent them from getting ill. There's no time in the schedule for illness.

The fitter you are when shooting a movie, the more enjoyable it's going to be. The last thing you want when undertaking one of these huge productions is to feel exhausted every single day because, as soon as you stop feeling capable, your confidence takes a hit. You'll be turning up for work every day in a far less confident mindset and that can be picked up on screen.

For much of Bryce's pre-production programme, I was in Britain and she was in America, so I trained her virtually. That worked well, as I had been in her gym before and I knew my way around it and what equipment she had. She would set up her phone on a tripod so I could see exactly what she was doing and I did the same while I demonstrated the exercises. She was also very committed to working virtually, showing the enthusiasm that she would have had if I had actually been in the gym with her. As the trainer, when you've got someone that keen, it makes the whole process much easier.

This is an example of a legs-specific workout that I put together for Bryce to improve her strength and conditioning. It was part of a complete fitness programme that also included upper-body-strength sessions, as well as dynamic yoga moves and a sprinkling of Pilates. People are always talking about aesthetic, but I wasn't thinking about that at all with Bryce – that wasn't our goal. I wanted to make her capable of performing in the film, and any change in how her legs looked was just a by-product of her improved strength and conditioning. I trained Bryce consistently for around six months before the shoot, and she was able to do everything that was asked of her in the stunt room and on the stage.

ACTIVATION AND CARDIO

I felt it was appropriate that the activation for *Jurassic World* was animalistic – Bryce did bear crawls, side crab walks and yoga moves such as cobra and downward dog. Her activation was dynamic to ger her body moving and flowing. For her cardio, Bryce would row, run and go on the bike, as well as doing plyometrics.

BRYCE'S 5–2 WORKOUT

DOUBLE BAND WORK

I started with this exercise because it's a little more simplistic than the others. That meant I could chat with Bryce while she did it, which helped me to gauge how she was feeling that day. I like bands as they allow you to have a smooth, constant tension on the muscle group.

- Put one band around your ankles and one band just above your knees.
- First move laterally, with your knees slightly soft or bent. Take ten steps to one side and then ten steps back.
- Go straight into a box. Your left leg goes forward first and then your right leg goes forward with your feet shoulder-width apart.
- Bend down into a squat position, with your knees slightly soft or bent. One foot goes out to the side, probably about 10 inches into a small squat, and then back to the beginning. Do ten on one side and then ten on the other.

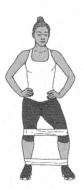 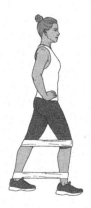

BOSU GOBLET SQUATS

If Bryce was going to be wearing high heels while running away from a T-Rex, she was going to need excellent stability and she got that from this exercise.

- Step onto the BOSU ball with the hard side up and your feet shoulder-width apart while holding a kettlebell or dumbbell in a cradle position close to your chest.
- Perform a conventional squat in which you're squatting down until your knees are at 90 degrees.
- Squeeze all the relevant muscle groups.
- Return to the start position while maintaining soft knees.

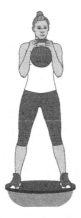
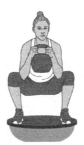

BOSU SPRINTER LUNGES

This exercise creates instability using the BOSU ball with the hard side up. It's always a great progression from conventional floor-based exercises.

- With the BOSU hard side up, put one foot in the middle while the other leg is parallel behind you. Your fingers are touching either side of the BOSU as if you are in a sprinting position.
- Drive the rear leg through, raise yourself to standing and elevate your knee in the air, so you're now standing on one leg.
- Return to the start position where your leg is directly behind you and your fingers are again touching the BOSU.

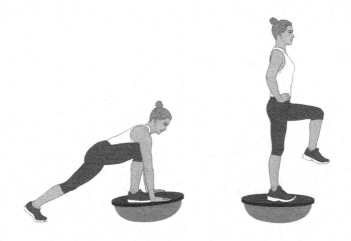

BOSU STEPOVERS

This exercise – which you do using the BOSU with the soft side up – is fantastic for lateral movement and for creating ballistic movement. Because it helps to raise your heart rate, it has a cardiovascular factor, too. It also allows your body to move from side to side, which is great for creating a more diverse action.

- The BOSU is soft side up. Stand by the side of it and put one foot in the middle.
- Skip over to the other side, replacing the foot on the BOSU with the other.
- As your foot lands on the other side, go into a slight squat.
- Skip back to the other side.
- Do this rhythmically with clenched hands out in front of you and your chest quite high.

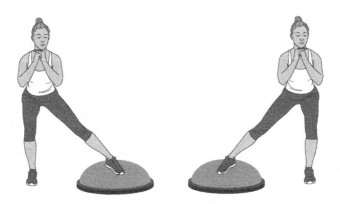

BURPEES WITH A JUMP

This exercise has stuck with me since my military days. I remember how brutal it could sometimes be, but it's also very dynamic. Quickly getting up off the ground and back onto your feet is extremely helpful in the movie-making business as you're asked to do that a lot. At the end of the movement, I asked Bryce to clap her hands above her head and shout out something funny. The clapping and shouting were introduced to inject a bit of humour into the session. It also made it easier for me to count the reps.

- Stand with your feet shoulder-width apart, and then squat down until your palms touch the floor.
- Your legs shoot out together at the same time behind you.
- Bring your legs back quickly, knees to chest, and then start to stand up before jumping in the air.
- Clap above your head.
- Return to the squat position.

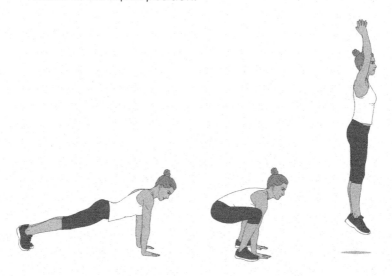

BRYCE'S WORKOUT

Double band work x 25 reps

Cardio

Double band work x 20 reps
BOSU goblet squats x 20 reps

Cardio

Double band work x 15 reps
BOSU goblet squats x 15 reps
BOSU sprinter lunges x 15 reps on each leg

Cardio

Double band work x 10 reps
BOSU goblet squats x 10 reps
BOSU sprinter lunges x 10 reps on each leg
BOSU stepovers x 10 reps on each leg

Cardio

Double band work x 8 reps
BOSU goblet squats x 8 reps
BOSU sprinter lunges x 8 reps on each leg
BOSU stepovers x 8 reps on each leg
Burpees with a jump x 8 reps

Cardio

PART 2

RECOVERY

10 | RECOVERY IS JUST AS IMPORTANT AS TRAINING

Many of us put almost all of the emphasis on our training when, in actual fact, recovery is just as important when it comes to fitness. If you don't recover, you don't make progress. Ensuring that your recovery programme is as competent as your training programme will allow you to do that.

Chris Pratt is an example of an actor who fully understands this. When I was preparing him for *Guardians of the Galaxy* and for the Jurassic World films, I saw how perfectly in tune he is with his training and recovery. He very obviously listens to his body and appreciates that you can't keep on pushing, especially when you're working long hours and doing short, sharp, intense workouts. I was really impressed that he was able to recognize that, and how keen he was to implement a solid recovery programme that allowed him to work and train again.

With other clients, who perhaps don't have that sporting background, I've had to educate them more on the value of recovery programmes. When I was training John Boyega for *Star Wars*, for instance, we really worked on this a lot, and I think he came away from those films with a very practical understanding of what sportspeople come up against all the time in the athletic world, and that what ultimately matters isn't how much you work or how hard you work, but how well you recover.

The faster and more efficiently you can recover, the better you're going to feel the next day. Your workout is a catalyst for the production of toxins and acids. When you're training efficiently in the right zone, your body can cope and can flush the toxins out. But once you start to overload and work beyond your capabilities, you will make more of them, and the body will struggle to get rid of them. They will sit in muscle tissue, causing soreness. It's normal for the body to produce toxins and acids – but what's important is being able to deal with them. If you can become more knowledgeable and efficient at dispersing these chemicals, using a variety of recovery methods, you're going to be ready to go again. Recovery is key to having a sustainable fitness programme.

I would ensure that Daniel Craig would have one day of 'pure recovery' a week during his programme for *No Time to Die*. When he was filming scenes in Scotland for the film, it was particularly physical. He was doing lots of running on uneven ground, which made it even more important to get the balance of recovery right.

In this part of the book, I'm going to be sharing my experience about the best way to recover, including trying to speed up the body's natural processes, and why, at the same time as training like a child, you ought to be recovering like a grandparent. There's also an entire section on sleep here, as I believe that it's the most important recovery tool of all – if you are sleeping well, you're probably going to recover well, too. I believe that recovery drills and treatments benefit your mind as well as your body, because while you're helping your body to heal, you're also ridding yourself of any mental fatigue.

BUILDING IN RECOVERY

You wouldn't skip a workout, so don't skip a recovery session. Even though you may feel fine right now, you still need to recover properly – it's an integral part of your programme. Ideally, you should never consciously feel as though you need to do something to recover. It should just be a natural part of your programme.

When preparing actors for films, recovery is always a prevention tool and I feel you should take the same approach. There's no point waiting to be sore before you start thinking about recovery: you should try to stop that soreness from happening in the first place. Prevention is key. If there's an option to have some treatment or some time to stretch or meditate, you should take it, regardless of whether you think you need it or not. You're not just looking at a short-term goal. This is to maintain your long-term objectives; it's all about combating and reducing the risks of fatigue and injuries that will hopefully never happen.

Recovery is the best way to end the week and ensures you are at your optimum and ready for the next seven days. But it doesn't have to be a Sunday – you can be flexible with when you do it. If you're bouncing around and feeling full of energy on the day you had been planning to do your recovery session, you could do a full workout instead.

Equally, if you're not 100 per cent ready for a workout session – perhaps your body's not quite right physically or you have a bit of mental fatigue – then have the courage and conviction (without feeling any guilt) to switch to a recovery session. This is all about intelligent fitness. Everything should be flexible, and you should never be restricted by your programme if you're not in the mood at a particular time. It's very easy to shift your recovery sessions around, just as long as you do them. Make the most of the strengths of the day and how you're feeling.

ACTIVE RECOVERY

You should view recovery as a workout. It's not a case of doing nothing. Active recovery is about doing something beneficial and diverse to complement what you would usually do in a training session. That could be dynamic yoga or swimming, a bike ride with the family, or playing some tennis or golf. Do something that takes you out of your normal range and mindset, giving you some escapism. Nine times out of ten, it's best to be outdoors for active recovery, which offers natural distractions, fresh air and stimulus.

You might be wondering why I don't recommend having a sedentary day of sitting around the house. The reason is that I don't think it's essential, physically or mentally, just to shut everything down. Active recovery helps to keep the body and the mind flowing, and you're also elevating your heart rate a little, which keeps you feeling alive. Allow yourself an athlete's nap on a Sunday afternoon (there's more on napping in the next chapter), but mainly just get out there and do some active recovery. It's a way of scheduling some fun time.

For us land-based creatures, being in water can sometimes feel like an alien environment, but that's why it provides such great escapism and therapy. In my view, from a mental standpoint, water is phenomenal. You're giving the body a diverse environment. When you're in the pool, the water is offsetting bodyweight. For instance, if you are in up to your waist, the water is bearing 50 per cent of your bodyweight. And if you are up to your chest it's about 75 per cent, rising to 80-90 per cent when you're up to your shoulders. It's the closest many of us will ever get to feeling weightless. When you're in water, you can jump up and down on your big toe, which you could never do on the street. Water can destress your body and give you a great sense of wellbeing.

When you move in the pool, you experience the resistance of being in the water but without overloading the muscles. That gives you the capability to move sore muscles and joints. This also makes the pool a great place for rehabilitation as it's a safe environment for injured muscles and joints. Equally, you can enjoy the benefits of the water pressure that helps to reduce any swelling and provides a small degree of pain relief. You're essentially taking the pressure off the body. In my opinion, the pool is the most useful recovery space. Using the water as resistance, you can do high-intensity drills with low impact, so you can increase your heart rate without the risk of hurting yourself. Spending time in the pool can result in a faster recovery and is also good for rehabilitation, which is what I did with Daniel Craig when he was injured.

SPEED UP THE PROCESS

There are a lot of old-school rules about having to wait a certain amount of time for recovery, which comes primarily from sleep and nutrition. But I would like to help you speed up the process using a variety of methods, so you can get on with feeling fresher with more energy to really maximize the benefits of your next session. You should never feel as though you want to take a week off, or even longer, to recover. When you have the balance right, your workout sessions should be energy-providing and not energy-depleting. I believe the main priority is to quickly reduce any swelling and soreness or lactic acid (which can cause delayed onset muscle soreness), as well as to relieve pain and tension.

I don't believe in 'no pain, no gain' or using pain as a metric for whether you're making gains. It only inhibits your progress. It's all about putting the right structures in place to achieve the best natural recovery possible. It often comes down to personal preference and what makes you feel good and gives you a sense of recuperation. Some therapies or aids are merely placebos, but they still have benefits. As with everything else in this book, you need to discover what works for you, but here are some of the treatments that I've used with my clients. I like to split the recovery process into three different groups:

- External and prescribed therapies
- Technological recovery aids
- Cold-water therapy

EXTERNAL THERAPIES

The hands-on treatment that a masseur, osteopath or chiropractor provides will not only benefit you from a recovery point of view, but also in terms of taking preventative measures. Most therapists will help you with diagnostics, identifying a future problem, injury or imbalance. They will feel, see and identify issues that you're not aware of yourself. While a masseur focuses on soft-tissue work, including reducing the swelling and removing the toxins, they can also help with relaxation and resetting the mind, as well as diagnostic prevention (identifying and addressing anything which could otherwise have become an issue in the future). An osteopath primarily works around the spine, but also helps with mobility and matters concerning the correct functioning of joints, as well as manipulation and soft-tissue work. A chiropractor focuses on joint manipulation and release.

Engaging the services of these types of professionals may seem like a bit of an indulgent thing to do if you've not considered it before in your fitness journey, but there really is no better way of addressing and correcting any potential issues before they become a greater problem. An objective opinion and human interaction for recovery can be most beneficial.

Getting treatments is key for most actors, but especially on athletic film productions. When working with actors on very physical films with a heavy workload, which may involve carrying weapons and equipment – such as with Charlize Theron on *The Old Guard* and Natalie Portman on *Annihilation* – having treatments on hand was critical for their recovery.

If you don't feel inclined to spend money on external treatment, another great method I can recommend is doing a complete session of dynamic stretching, featuring ten exercises and ten reps of each. Dynamic stretching encourages blood flow into the muscle group you're targeting, opens up fibres and can help remove toxins, which can alleviate soreness and aid your recovery. Depending on how much time you have, you could go through the whole routine once or twice. This is one of my favourite sessions to do at the end of the week (look up the explanations of these dynamic stretching exercises in the Activation and Deactivation chapter on page 43).

- Bear crawl into pigeon
- Narrow squat into side abductor stretch
- Reverse lunge with hip flexor stretch
- Adapted mountain climber with hamstring activation
- Regular sit-up with lumbar twist
- Kneeling to standing with foot stretch into child's pose
- Quad stretch reverse lunge knee pull
- Side spider crawl
- Pedal to standing
- Plank to pike into cobra

TECHNOLOGICAL RECOVERY AIDS

From contactless percussion tools to electrical stimulation, I use a variety of different technologies with actors and I encourage you to try some of them. Some of the equipment is pricey, but you could look at hiring those aids for a short period rather than buying them.

CONTACTLESS PERCUSSION TOOLS

When working with actors who need help with their recovery, I regularly use these fast and effective tools which are shaped like guns or drills, with vibrating rollers and balls on the ends. They relax the muscles and increase blood flow, with all its healing properties, to different parts of the body.

Contactless percussion tools help to get rid of lactic acid and any other toxins in the body. While they may be on the expensive side, using them is a non-intrusive and very effective, efficient way to speed up the recovery process and to prevent injuries. I often turn to such tools on set as they can be operated while the actors are still in costume, which means it doesn't cause a delay and you get straight into the area that you're trying to treat. They are also easy to carry around in your bag and can be used either before or after a workout or even during a session (see Harrison Ford's *Indiana Jones* workout on page 159).

ELECTRICAL STIMULATION AIDS

These types of aids, which include Compex TENS machines, provide electrical stimulation to targeted muscles. They are often used in the early stages of rehab to attract blood flow and to help prevent muscle wastage – when the muscle tissue isn't being used and it starts to weaken – without using resistance. They enable a muscle to recover while allowing a joint to be stimulated. They can also act as a pump mechanism to drain away any excessive swelling. They are often used in conjunction with ice and compression to speed up recovery.

Of course, some of these pieces of kit I use with my clients aren't cheap, and I appreciate that not everyone will want to invest in a TENS machine or similar. But they are incredibly effective and worth knowing about. A lot of these machines are available for hire, which might make more sense if it's not something you need to use regularly.

Something worth looking into is a NormaTec, a massage tool that works on air pressure. It's like putting on inflatable trousers as it uses compartmentalized air pressure, making it an effective post-workout recovery aid. The pressure helps ease muscle ache and also increases circulation in the affected areas. NormaTec is portable and you can lie on your bed or sit in a chair and instantly start recovering. It also works on a very simple, computerized system that allows you to control the pressure and the time. You can even fall asleep while you have it on. It's a great device if you want to multitask during your recovery, such as reading a script or a book. I use this system a lot when I have several actors needing to recover at the same time and I only have one pair of hands.

Another high-tech piece of kit that could also be hired rather than bought is AlterG, a revolutionary rehab tool designed by NASA that has the same physiological effects as water displacement. It's basically a giant air bubble on top of a treadmill, which can take some of your weight, and can be adjusted to make you lighter or heavier. That means you can gently load an injury while allowing you to get back to more of a natural movement and walking pattern. You can decrease the percentage of bodyweight that the bubble is compensating for until eventually you're back to 100 per cent capability.

COLD-WATER THERAPY

Cold water is believed to have great healing properties. During a shoot in Ireland, I remember going to a place called Forty Foot where people swim in the sea throughout the year and submerge themselves while the icy waves crash around them. I chatted with the swimmers, who couldn't speak highly enough of the mental and physical benefits of cold-water swimming on a daily basis. They said it gave them increased clarity, focus and energy. For some, it even offered pain relief. When you lower yourself into cold water, it's a massive shock at first. It's horrendous, in fact. But if you can persevere, you'll soon be hooked – I think people almost get addicted to bathing in it. They do it every day and can't live without it. That's a healthy addiction to have as it will boost your immune system by stimulating the production of more white blood cells, while also reducing the toxins in your body, as the heart pumps more blood and that helps to flush them away.

You could also expose yourself to cold water by getting into a bathtub filled with cold water and ice. At the other end of the scale are cryotherapy chambers. A couple of minutes of standing in extreme temperatures – the chamber can be minus 100 degrees Celsius or even colder – can help to activate your body's recovery systems. I've used this therapy a lot with actors, including with Daniel during his preparation for the Bond films.

For more isolated cold therapy, I like a system called Game Ready, a computerized cryotherapy machine which allows you to apply compression and ice to an area of the body to aid recovery. I've tried it with actors and also on myself – you can even use it when you're sleeping. If you don't have access to that piece of kit, the old-school method of ice in a bag or a bag of frozen peas will create similar effects by helping to reduce swelling and offer pain relief.

PLUNGE POOLS

Daniel would often go in and out of hot and cold plunge pools, with three minutes in hot water and then three in cold water. It's great for boosting your immune system, as well for aiding your recovery and wellbeing. When you go into the cold pool, blood vessels close to the skin constrict. And then when you are in the hot pool, the blood vessels open up and more blood flows through them, helping to flush out toxins. If you don't have access to plunge pools, you could create your own version of hot and cold therapy by getting into a warm bath first and then placing ice on a sore or injured part of your body for ten to fifteen minutes (don't put the ice directly onto your skin, but rather wrap it in a tea towel). Then submerge the affected area in the warm water again. Do two or three rounds of that.

11 | BECOME A PERFORMANCE SLEEPER

Sleep can provide the best indication of how you are performing within your programme. When your training, nutrition and other elements of your recovery are balanced, that is reflected in the quality of your sleep. If one of those elements is too extreme or off somehow, I find that sleep patterns are affected detrimentally. If your workouts are too intense or your nutrition is too strict, that will certainly have an impact on how you're sleeping.

I'm always asking my clients about their sleep. In pre-production or on set during the shoot, it tends to be the first thing I talk to them about in the morning when we meet up. Sleep is the most powerful recovery tool you have. I think many of us underestimate the importance of good sleep, but it's probably the biggest factor in the recovery process as you're never going to make any gains if you're not getting quality sleep. Your body heals itself when it's asleep as it's releasing HGH (human growth hormone), which is essential for repair and rejuvenation, and helps you to perform the next day.

If you have had a poor night of broken sleep, you're likely to feel low on energy and that could lead to a higher risk of injury because your concentration won't be at optimum levels. When you're tired and lacking in energy, there's a greater chance that you'll start to crave non-essential energy providers like sugar, and that will disturb your nutrition plan.

Of course, sleep works the other way too – if you sleep too much, your body and mind feel as though they are going into hibernation, and it becomes more difficult to get yourself going and motivated when you get up. It's about finding your own personal balance and what works for you and your energy levels. When you wake up naturally from uninterrupted sleep and have had at least four hours of REM – when you go into the deep reparative state that the body needs – that's a sure sign that you're on your way to becoming a performance sleeper. Your body will have fulfilled its duties of repair, reboot and regenerate within the sleep cycle.

TRACK YOUR SLEEP

Sleep is, of course, a very natural part of being alive. But some of us are much better at it than others, and if you're not a bad sleeper yourself, you're sure to know someone who is. If you can sleep anywhere, you're one of the lucky few – only a small percentage of people have that ability. Most of us need to have the right environment in order to enjoy a quality night's sleep. You need to create that environment; this takes a little conscious effort and maybe some experimentation to see what works for you. My routine includes having a shower right before going to bed, as I find it relaxing. Maybe there's something you need to do, which you hadn't considered before, that will allow you to have the best night's sleep?

If you're not sure what the best environment is for you, try keeping a sleep diary for a while until you discover which circumstances produce the best results – you might find it helpful to create a sleep grid for yourself like the one opposite. Log what you did on those days when you woke up and thought: 'Wow, I slept well and I feel great.' Record how many hours of sleep you had, the approximate time you went to sleep and the time you woke up, and what the environment was like. We all have a natural biorhythm – our body wants to shut down at a particular time for a certain number of hours. Things as simple as the temperature in the room can also make a key difference in determining whether we get quality sleep.

	1	2	3	4	5	6	7
What time did I go to bed?							
When did I fall asleep?							
What time did I wake up?							
Did I wake during the night?							
What did I do in the hour before going to bed?							
Was there anything different about my sleep environment?							
What did I eat during the day?							
How did I feel in the morning?							

Performance sleep is created through your environment. Do you need a light on in the room? Or is total darkness with blackout curtains blocking out the street lights an absolute must? Do you prefer complete quiet at night, or soft music, or are you used to ambient sounds such as the low rumble of traffic? What else is going on in the room? Do you like to sleep with the window open in order to feel fresh air on your face? What are the sensory elements that give you your optimum sleep? Once you have worked this out, try to set those environmental factors in place before you get into bed.

Conversely, if you've had a bad night's sleep, make a note of whether there was anything different about the environment, as that could help you spot a pattern. That could be a particular food that affects your sleep, or drinking too much liquid, or something as simple as comfort. A great many people sleep on the wrong mattresses for their body type, and don't have the right pillows for their necks, shoulders and backs. These are very common problems with very easy solutions.

In an ideal world, you won't be stimulating your brain with a screen for at least an hour before bed, and your phone will be on silent, but I'm a realist and I appreciate that this won't always be possible. I understand you might need or like to be on your laptop just before you sleep, or you might be on your phone contacting family and friends. But if you're serious about performance, you will find a way to minimize your exposure to screens before you go to sleep.

Stimulants, such as coffee and tea, and drinks that are high in sugar are probably going to hinder your sleep. I know that everyone has a different lifestyle and outlook, and can get stimulated by different things, so decide what works for you. Using technology to measure sleeping patterns is now really popular. We use tech to monitor our workouts and so if sleep is part of your performance, why not monitor that as well?

TUNE YOUR NUTRITION

If your sleep patterns are suffering, it's a sign that something is out of balance. If you're feeling hunger pangs or are bloated, you'll find it hard to relax and get into that meditative state which leads to quality sleep. When people are on a stricter nutrition plan, they often feel as though they want to get as much sleep as possible because they think that will allow them to get rid of their cravings, and so they go to bed earlier. But that usually doesn't work as this course of action won't produce good-quality sleep. Quite the opposite, in fact.

If my clients tell me they are sleeping badly, I'll try to tailor their programme to ensure they get enough sleep and of a decent standard. That could be something as simple as slightly lowering the intensity of the workout or reducing or adding calories to create a better balance for them. To avoid waking up in the middle of the night feeling hungry, you could try having a snack before you go to bed. Of course, it's important to eat the right thing at this time of the day – for example, I wouldn't eat meat too late as there's a chance that it could give you reflux. Instead, I would suggest having a snack that feels more therapeutic and is easier to digest – something like a soup or a broth, which will give you a little bit of hydration and can also contain different food groups. You could have an anti-inflammatory element, such as turmeric, as well as minerals, such as magnesium or zinc, to help put you in a more relaxed state. These late-night snacks may involve a little trial and error to work out which is the most beneficial. It's about fine-tuning what you're eating and discovering what satisfies you the most at that particular time.

You could even try a 'sleepy' tea, such as camomile, before bed, though I think the effects may be more mental than physiological. The process of making the tea before bed – even the smell of it brewing – will become a signal to the body that it needs to get ready for sleep by relaxing and slowing down. The body loves patterns and sequences, and it will start to recognize when you're getting ready for bed.

BEDTIME

Everyone's body clock is different, so make sure you listen to yours. When does your body start to slow and shut down and prepare to fall asleep? Ensure you tune in to your body's natural biorhythm and if you're feeling sleepy, don't try to fight it – go to bed earlier. Equally, there's no point in trying to go to sleep at 9 p.m. if you're unlikely to achieve deep sleep until midnight. You might as well go to bed later.

Always pay attention to what your body is telling you and work out when you should go to bed to have the optimum sleep. The body loves consistency and eventually it will create a natural pattern and behaviour at the same time each day. If you can get into a regular routine of going to bed at a particular time, that will help you to get good-quality sleep.

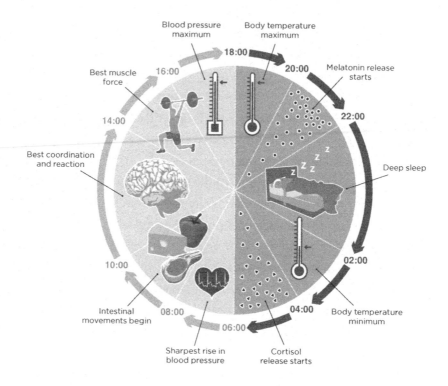

While on production, actors notoriously get up very early. It's not unusual to get picked up at 4.30 a.m. in order arrive on set by 6 a.m. – which could allow time for a workout, activation and breakfast – and then deal with hair, make-up and costume before walking through the stage door to start work around 9 a.m. When you've got an early start like this, you need to adjust your regular bedtime to ensure you get enough sleep. Don't think that you can survive on fewer hours of sleep than normal, as that will have a detrimental effect on your performance, concentration levels and overall wellbeing: everyone's mood is worse when they haven't had enough sleep.

THE MAGIC NUMBER

Everyone's sleep requirements are different. Many people need eight hours of sleep a night, while some require six hours and others can get by with four. What matters is the quality of your sleep and how you feel when you get up in the morning.

Sometimes we sleep for a long time, but this might only be superficial sleep, and we haven't entered into the deep sleep mode, the period when the body slows down with a lower heart rate and lower metabolism, allowing the brain to switch to sorting and storing the information from the previous day. That's when you get quality sleep. I always say to my clients that it's much better to have four hours of deep sleep than to have eight hours of superficial sleep. It takes a while for you to get into that deep reparative state when everything is being rebooted ready for the next day. You won't get the deep sleep that you need if, for example, you've been drinking alcohol, as alcohol is essentially a sedative and results in the suppression of REM sleep for a lot of the night. You'll know if you've had enough deep sleep based on how you feel when you wake up. If you've only had superficial sleep, you'll still be tired, but if you've had enough deep sleep, you'll feel rejuvenated and ready for the day ahead.

Too much sleep is not good either, as that can have a detrimental effect on how you feel the next morning because it throws off your biological clock. If you wake up around the time you do most mornings and then decide that you're going to go back to sleep again, it's like starting and then quickly shutting down an engine. It's better to have the optimum amount of sleep and then get up straight away rather than snoozing for too long.

TRAINING AND SLEEP

If your sessions are running late into the evening, you're going to be raising your heart rate and metabolism, and then your body needs enough time to stabilize itself before it can begin to relax and get into the right state for sleep. As a general rule, try to ensure that your workout ends at least two hours before you go to bed. I've changed the times of my clients' workouts, moving them to earlier in the day to help them improve their sleep. I also prefer to have a liquid post-workout meal as it can be more easily digested, which should contribute to a better night's sleep.

I often encourage my clients to take the opportunity to have what I call an 'athlete's nap', which allows them to quickly reboot and recharge. When they get a short break on a movie set, perhaps when stages or lighting are being changed, or if there's a technical issue, this is valuable downtime. That's when actors might put their feet up and have a nap.

Having an 'athlete's nap' is an art and not a science; you have to find out what works for you. However, I don't recommend napping for longer than twenty minutes, as you don't want to compromise your energy and sabotage your nightly sleep. If you doze for too long, your body will think that it's about to go into a deep sleep and then it takes too long to start it up again after waking. If you can nap for up to twenty minutes it's almost like a form of meditation, and you give your body and mind a little bit of a rest, reset and reboot. You can then get on with the rest of the day with more energy, and even greater focus and concentration.

Many of us worry about sleeping badly, and unfortunately that's probably the worst thing you can do. Have the confidence to know that we're all capable of getting a restful night, and that there are lots of factors at play that are within your control. You have to find a way of discovering your perfect sleep patterns. That's often where keeping a sleep diary comes in. Or sometimes it's as simple as taking some time away – checking into a hotel or staying with a friend for a couple of nights – as breaking a pattern of poor sleep by changing your environment can be really effective.

12 | MANAGING INJURIES AND SETBACKS

In his foreword, Daniel Craig writes about how I would help 'repair' him after he sustained injuries or experienced inevitable physical setbacks on a Bond set. But physically repairing someone who's been injured is only one part of recovery, as a person's mental health can also be affected unless you have a constructive plan and a clear path to recovery. It's easy to feel down after getting injured, as the healing process can be very frustrating. I discovered this myself recently while writing this book, when I broke my ankle.

Managing the mental and emotional fallout of an injury is often harder than dealing with the physical side and rehabilitation. In fact, it plays a significant part in my job, no more so than when I was working alongside Daniel during his Bond movies. Just as athletes at the top of their game get injured when they're constantly pushing their bodies to the limit, Daniel hurt various parts of his body while performing action scenes, including damaging his ankle while filming *No Time to Die*. No matter who you are, you will feel vulnerable when you've been physically impaired. I've found that all setbacks have solutions and part of my job is to manage my clients back to full health in the most efficient way without cutting corners.

INJURIES ARE INEVITABLE

Injuries happen. They're practically inescapable if you're filming action movies. I've had to accept that. Avoiding injuries is, of course, my primary goal when working with actors. For prevention, I would look at the stunt sequences for a Bond film and see what they were asking Daniel's body to do. When I thought the sequence was going to be hard and there was going to be impact on his knees and elbows, for instance, I would try to protect and support those parts of the body by taping, as well as using pads for protection under the costume. But, for all the safety and prevention I can provide when actors are filming a chase sequence or other athletic stunt sequences, there has to be some kind of realism otherwise it simply won't look authentic.

The big stunt sequences were rehearsed so many times. But it always felt different when they were actually being filmed. Daniel would have rehearsed a scene in loose workout gear and trainers, but for filming he would have been wearing a tailored suit and possibly dress shoes as well. He might have been running across an uneven surface, carrying a weapon, with explosions going off all around him. When Daniel had 400 crew and three cameras pointing at him on set, he adopted a different feel and mindset compared to that of the rehearsal environment. His adrenaline level was higher, his motivation and speed were increased, and after doing several takes he would also have been dealing with lactic acid and fatigue.

I can still clearly remember all those moments when Daniel injured himself during filming. When shooting *Quantum of Solace*, he hurt his shoulder while doing a stunt in a falling plane. I recall the time he tore both calf muscles on *Skyfall*. And there was the moment when Daniel was involved in a fight scene for *Spectre* – inside a train at Pinewood Studios – and he injured the anterior cruciate ligament in his knee, which I then had to manage for the rest of the shoot. There were other smaller setbacks, too.

The body is a complex, funny thing. It's sometimes not the big things that trip you up and hinder you. It's also the small, less athletic issues that no amount of health and safety checks could have avoided, such as slipping on the street or missing a step.

While you probably won't be doing anything as risky as shooting an action movie, you have to prepare yourself for the possibility that you're going to experience a setback at some stage. Accepting this in advance will make things easier to cope with when it happens; it won't come as a massive shock.

KEEP TRAINING THE REST OF YOUR BODY

Within a couple of weeks of Daniel's ankle injury on *No Time to Die*, I encouraged him to get back into the gym to manage and work around it, including training his upper body. After the operation, I tried to quickly figure out the path to his continuing to train physically and to stay mentally engaged while following the protocol and rehabilitation of that injury.

Many people become sedentary while recovering from injury but, in my opinion, you should continue training the rest of your body whenever possible. I believe you will benefit from keeping your body and brain engaged, especially as working out will encourage the release of crucial chemicals and hormones that will help the body to repair itself. If you can keep the body moving and in its most natural state – including maintaining metabolism – it will accelerate the healing process courtesy of increased circulation. Inactivity can shut down muscles, which can lead to tissue atrophy. Injuries are only a temporary setback, not a full body shutdown. Maintaining your bodily training also prevents your physicality from sliding. Keep your body ticking over and doing all the things that it would normally do.

Every time an actor is injured, I sit down with them and devise a programme to work around their limitations and put the body into a happy healing state. That can include making sure the nutrition is right, such as shifting to a more anti-inflammatory plan (see the nutrition section in Part Three for more on anti-inflammatories). I am always investigating how they can best recover and return to 100 per cent capacity. By carrying on with training the rest of your body, you're also distracting yourself from the injury and allowing yourself to focus on something else for a while. Daniel and I decided we would do whatever we could to work around that ankle injury so that as soon as it was healed, he would be in great shape and ready to get on with the rest of the shoot.

LISTEN TO YOUR EMOTIONS

With most injuries, you can see the physical effects due to swelling or bruising. But what you also need to monitor is the invisible secondary factor – how the injury is impacting on your mental health. One sign that you're not doing too well is when you lose interest in your rehab and the things you need to do to heal your body. Injuries are notoriously frustrating. As the body takes time to heal itself naturally, the simple and practical things in life become more difficult.

Injuries are even more challenging for someone who is used to being very physical, and who can no longer do all that they used to. During such times, take the opportunity to learn about yourself. You need to be able to differentiate between the days when it's just a case of not having slept that well and you're experiencing frustrations, and the moments when it seems more serious and you're feeling down, and you can't snap out of it. When you're injured, you should give as much focus to the mental side as the physical.

If you have a long-term injury, I believe you will almost always come out the other side both physically and mentally stronger. Dealing with an injury is a form of mental conditioning as you're proving to yourself what you're capable of during the recovery process. While you will naturally become mentally stronger, you can enhance that process by resetting your goals. Set yourself new challenges for when the injury has healed. And remind yourself that what matters is not the way you enter into something, but the way you come out of it.

You have ups and downs with your fitness, just like anything in life. You have to relish the positive moments and also learn how to manage the negative times by finding your trigger for working out how to escape them. I think we probably learn more when we're down than when we're up. You don't have to talk yourself down, but you do sometimes have to talk yourself up.

Everyone has rough days when they're injured or have setbacks. Don't be afraid of voicing your feelings and saying that you're not up for something. Sometimes we just need to recognize that it's OK to feel down and it's impossible to be upbeat all the time. Don't fight your emotions; they're there, whether we like it or not, and it's how we deal with them that's important. It's always good to have some go-to activities that snap you out of dwelling on your injury or the fact that you can't follow your normal training programme for a few days. It might be music or a TV show that distracts you, or going for a coffee or walking the dog; anything that gives you some distraction and some time out of the house is great.

SET A PATH BACK TO NORMALITY

When you have a setback or injury, there's nothing more important than having a plan to help bring you back to normality. If you don't have a plan, you'll go insane, frustrated by having no sense of when you'll return to full health again. You need to have goals, micro goals and moments of progression that you can tick off along the way, as this provides the mental momentum that you need to make headway. If there's a set programme, you will have an idea of where you need to be in week one, how things will look in week two, how active you'll be in week three, and so on.

It's tough when you have an injury for the first time as you don't know what the time frame for recovery is or how long it will take your body to naturally heal. If you haven't been through that situation before, it feels like you might never be OK again and it can be difficult when you don't have any previous experience to draw on.

I surround myself with a great team of professionals who offer expert medical advice, providing me with the tools and information to help my clients and keep us on the right path. If you can, stay engaged with your medical professional – perhaps your physio or your doctor – and discuss how long they estimate it will take for your body to heal itself. Also ask them when you can move on to the next part of the process, as everyone's healing time is different.

DON'T TRY TO COPE ON YOUR OWN

As a trainer, I'm primarily a motivator, and that goes for injury time, too. I'm here to keep actors engaged. When anyone is feeling down because of an injury, it's my job to reassure them that they will survive it. I show them that they're making incremental progress with their rehab and fitness and they'll be on the right track to being in great shape again soon. I tell them: 'You're here, you're in it, and you need to do this the best way you can. There is no point focusing on the ifs, buts and maybes – only focus on I did, I can, I will.'

It's inevitable when you work with people for long periods of time that you form a friendship, especially when you are dealing with their health and wellbeing as that's extremely personal. After five Bond movies, Daniel and I have developed a close relationship, though of course I have to differentiate between when I'm working and when I'm not. I'm professional while I'm on set and in that work environment but, outside of work, Daniel is also a friend and, like any friend, you support them when they experience setbacks.

I would suggest that you find someone you can chat to – maybe a friend or a family member, or perhaps someone who has been through a similar injury setback and made a full recovery. They can reassure you that you are making progress and there is some light at the end of the tunnel.

When I broke my ankle recently, which required an operation, Daniel was among the friends who messaged me, letting me know that he was supporting me through it. Out of all my friends, he had the greatest empathy as he had experienced the same thing. When you've been there – even if it's not exactly the same injury – you can also discuss the roadmap back to normality with someone who needs your help.

BE PATIENT

One of the biggest myths in fitness is that you need to push through pain. But that macho way of thinking, dismissing the pain and carrying on regardless, is dangerous. We now know that you don't have to be in pain to make gains. Of course, there are varying degrees of pain, and when you're pushing yourself in your recovery programme it's going to hurt, but you have to be able to differentiate between progressive pain and the damaging pain that can lead to setbacks.

For most people, it can be hard to know when to crack on with your rehab and when to rest and take it more slowly. The way I like to structure it is to have a care day, then a conditioning day and back to a care day again. If you just do a care day or just a conditioning day and then expect to recover quickly, it simply won't happen. You need a balance and I think you can achieve that by alternating between the two. If you're only conditioning, you won't be helping the injury – instead of addressing the problem, you could even be making it worse. Balance is key.

On the conditioning day, you should be doing specific exercises to strengthen joints or redevelop muscle that you have lost since the injury. You're trying to build strength, balance and mobility, and to restore your patterns and sequences. On the care day, I would talk to my physical therapist about whether I have had any reaction to the conditioning day and see if that allows me to move on. I call this process test, rest and progress. On a care day, you might have manual therapy, icing, flexing and stretching, and general rest.

When you're with someone for ten or twelve hours a day, and sometimes even longer, you get to know the signs of fatigue and when they're not fully engaged, and you also pick up on when they're unsure or not comfortable with something. After many years of working with Daniel, for example, I know his capabilities and I know when I can push him and when I can't. That comes from spending a lot of time with somebody on a daily basis.

As a trainer, this becomes a crucial part of your job. The most sensible approach is always to be cautious and not to try to accelerate the rehabilitation process. With experience gained over the years, you learn how to tread that fine line between accelerated progression and natural progression. If you push too hard, you risk setting the process back several weeks. Sometimes you have to let nature take its course. If you experience an adverse reaction, back off and go back to natural progression. Wait until that reaction has subsided and then try again with accelerated progression.

Sometimes, an injury is the body's way of saying that you're doing too much. If you hurt yourself by accident, of course, that's hard to avoid, but with an injury sustained during training it's a little bit more within your control. And if you do suffer such a setback, it's still an opportunity to learn more about your body and what works for you. Ask yourself whether you could be doing anything different with your workouts and nutrition to reduce the chance of it happening again. Or eliminate a particular exercise or training method which doesn't feel right, gives you pain or doesn't suit your biomechanics, which is how your body moves.

PART 3
NUTRITION

13 | FUEL YOUR BODY

The right nutrition will give you performance, provide energy and contribute to your mental health. There's so much emotion and psychology wrapped up in every mouthful, even in every sip of that recovery shake you have after your workout. Nutrition sets the tone for the day – your wellbeing, your recovery and your sleep all revolve around it. Our relationship with food – how we view it and what we use it for – are really important for our general health and, needless to say, the more you know, the more you can help fuel your body with what it needs. Good nutrition is simply about making informed decisions and avoiding bad habits.

Whether you're an actor or an athlete, or someone beginning their fitness journey, you're not going to achieve your goals if you're not eating the right things. You might be training hard, but if your nutrition is terrible you're not giving yourself the best chance of progression and you may struggle to maximize your genetic capability.

In this section of the book, I'm going to be sharing my thoughts and opinions on nutrition based on twenty-five years of experience and observation. I'll also explain why I feel deprivation is the very worst thing you can do with your consumption habits, and why I'm relaxed about the occasional glass of wine or beer. I believe you should be able to switch between two different mindsets – the one in which you're focused on 'performance nutrition' and the other that relates to mental wellness and social engagement with friends and family. This approach has certainly been successful for my clients. You'll see that I like to keep things fairly simple and I hope this chapter gives you the inspiration and insight you need to improve your nutrition and avoid ever having to go on a diet.

PERFORMANCE vs WELLNESS

Nutrition stimulates feelings. It also satisfies feelings, puts out fires and pacifies cravings. As soon as you understand what certain foods can do for you, you'll have a totally different relationship with nutrition.

Your view of food depends on what state or mode you're in. If you're injured, you should regard food as medicinal. When you're about to do some high-intensity activity, you'll see food as an energy provider, and afterwards you'll perceive it as an aid to your recovery. Food can also enhance sleep. Your perception of food is constantly changing. But inevitably your body will let you know what it requires, whether that's energy, repair or rest, depending on the circumstances. If you can switch between two different modes – the 'performance nutrition' mindset and the 'wellness' mindset – that creates great balance.

To get yourself into a performance nutrition mindset, it's helpful to think about what the nutrition is going to do for you and what the physiological effects of consuming that food will be. When you're working towards a fitness goal, there are going to be certain foods, drinks and supplement combinations that you will have before and after training to aid your performance. You need to consider what you're consuming and how that will provide you with stimulation and energy (whether for immediate use or stored for later). When I sit down to eat something, I'm always asking myself: 'What is this going to do for me and why am I having it now?'

There are also many types of nutritional combinations that you can consume before sleeping – such as a mineral with a protein –

which will help you to repair and then perform the next day.

While it's good to adopt that performance nutrition mindset, you have to be capable of switching out of it when you're with family and friends, and in more of a social environment. It can be helpful to think, 'OK, that was my performance nutrition, but this is now a social occasion and I'm enhancing my wellbeing through being looser with my nutrition and being around people I care about who aren't so conscious about what they're eating.' That's a completely different mindset. If you can easily transition from one to another when you need to, you'll have a much healthier relationship with food and will give yourself the best chance of achieving your fitness and nutritional goals.

DEPRIVATION CAN DESTROY EVERYTHING

There's nothing worse than someone who is feeling miserable on an overly strict nutrition plan (I'm trying to avoid using the word 'diet' here as I dislike it so much!). It's physically and mentally unsustainable, and as well as being awful for the individual in question, it's just as horrendous for everyone around them, as they have to put up with the ever-changing moods. Without a doubt, the biggest mistake you can make with your nutrition is to be too extreme and deprive yourself of the food groups that your body is used to.

In my experience, if you try to cut out an entire food group or start skipping meals, that does crazy things to the brain. You're starving yourself – the body and brain don't react well to extreme situations and will rebel against you. If you're too restrictive, you're guaranteed to be unhappy and you won't be able to sustain such a rigid programme.

If you tell yourself that you can't have a particular type of food, you will end up thinking about and craving that food all the time. Psychologically, I think it's so important to feel as though anything is on the table and that you can have whatever you want whenever you want it. Choice is essential, but you'll need to challenge yourself to stay in control by making informed decisions. When you're being restrictive, there's eventually nowhere to go, as you can't reduce your calories to zero, and that's never going to lead to a happy, healthy life.

All the actors I've worked with have healthy relationships with nutrition because I've arranged things that way with some help from chefs, such as Sarah Sugden, who prepare their food on set. I don't do restrictive. I don't do deprivation. Deprivation doesn't just damage your physical and mental wellbeing; it also destroys your metabolism and stalls your performance.

Never turn to deprivation to achieve an aesthetic. The body will go looking for energy from somewhere in order to fuel the performance that you want from it. It will start to go catabolic, using muscle tissue as energy, which means it's reducing your hard-won gains. That's why you won't get the performance you want if you're depriving yourself.

You certainly don't want your body to enter a state of shutdown or shock. If the body feels as though it's being deprived, it will always burn through muscle tissue ahead of fat. This is why putting the body in a comfort zone is much more beneficial when it comes to sustained fat-burning. Always work with your body and never against it. If you deprive yourself, you may look a little leaner but you could still have the same body-fat percentage because your muscle tissue has been reduced, and in the long run that will reduce your metabolism.

Quite simply, what all this boils down to is that if your output exceeds your input, through performance and not deprivation, you will achieve your athletic gains. You need to work out where your optimum zone is so you're not being deprived of essential nutrition. For athletes, nutrition is about consumption and never about nutritional restriction.

Restrictive nutrition can have many consequences. For example, if a woman deprives herself of the nutrition she needs for everyday life, her periods may stop and it could also result in hair loss, brittle nails, bad skin and premature ageing. That is too high a price for your aesthetic; always look at the bigger picture and always focus on your overall, long-term health.

If you put yourself on a restrictive plan, you will eventually suffer from a lack of energy, making illness and injury more likely. You're more susceptible to muscular or connective tissue injuries if you're not in an optimum, balanced state supported by good nutrition. If you're an actor, any day lost to injury or illness causes scheduling and financial problems for the production. But even if you're not in the film industry, you don't want to increase your chances of being ill or injuring yourself through restrictive nutrition in the hope that it might enhance your aesthetic.

Instead of focusing on the things you're going to cut from your diet, think about what you'll change and what you may add, such as more natural foods rather than processed. What has worked for me is introducing varied, good-quality food. Whatever you do, don't take a restrictive approach and impose that on anyone else. Don't be that person whom no one wants to invite to their home because they've become so difficult about what they will eat. Remember that everyone's relationship with food is different; don't imagine anyone else wants to follow the same nutrition plan you're on. Always maintain flexibility.

THEME DAYS

Throughout *No Time to Die*, Daniel Craig and I would have Vegetarian Mondays, Pescatarian Tuesdays, Vegan Wednesdays, White Meat Thursdays and Red Meat Fridays. Weekends would be based around social and family time. The idea behind the theme days is that you're setting daily parameters rather than being too restrictive, and it also allows for some variation – you shouldn't stick to eating the same thing all the time when there's so much choice available within your chosen themes.

Recently, I've gone a bit more plant-based. I was influenced by the time I spent preparing Woody Harrelson for *Star Wars*. He's a raw vegan and it was incredible to see how much energy he had. I feel as though we could all go that way a bit more, as there are a lot more plant-based performance foods and I'm realizing that in addition to the health benefits, the performance benefits are also just as good. However, this doesn't mean you have to cut out entire food groups (unless of course you're doing it for ethical, health or merely taste reasons). We could all eat more plants without labelling ourselves as vegetarian or vegan. It's great to have a foot in all camps, as then you can have a balanced diet. If you really want a name for yourself, you can always call yourself a 'flexitarian'.

I know other trainers suggest a 'cheat day' at the weekends, but I would suggest renaming that a 'choice day', because if you start talking about cheating it's only going to encourage you to deviate too much from your programme. After the weekend, you're back to your vegan or vegetarian theme day on Monday, which sets you back on your plan. In my experience, you're starting the week afresh and allowing your body to reset and reboot its systems.

I find it's easy to carry that theme around in your head, so if you're out and about and having to eat on the run during a busy day, it sets the parameters for what you can consume. But don't be too hard on yourself as, unless you have the perfect environment and structure around you, it's almost impossible to stick to it. It may well be that on a day when you were supposed to be having a pescatarian theme day, all that was available was red meat. But that's fine as with theme days you have the flexibility of making everything interchangeable. You could swap two around so you're still doing each one once in a week. It's easy to stick to these five parameters rather than hard and fast meal plans. Within those themes, you also need to look at your 'macros' – the percentage of your calories that come from either protein, carbohydrates or good fats. The percentages are determined by your goals and the mode you're trying to put your body in, for example whether you're building muscle tissue (increase your protein) or you want more energy (up your carbohydrates).

QUALITY PROTEIN FOR BUILD MODE

In the first few weeks, it wasn't easy ensuring that Chris Evans had the right amount of nutrition when training for *Captain America*. When I met him, foot-long meatball subs were a particular favourite of his. Chris was always on the move, and he would often just grab whatever was to hand. Soon enough, though, he was eating the necessary nutrition to supplement his training and improve his health. One of my challenges was getting him to consume enough protein to gain muscle mass, but also stopping him from storing excess calories or energy as fat cells. Between prescribed meals, Chris had fast-acting protein shakes to aid recovery plus a slow-release, pre-sleep protein shake, and he also snacked on fruit, nuts and seeds.

Protein is key for repairing the muscle tissue you have damaged while training. It's all about feeding that muscle as it grows, adapts and gets stronger. You simply can't be in calorie deficit – when you use more calories than you're eating – through this process.

Think of muscle tissue as an engine burning up calories. Every pound of muscle requires around thirty calories a day just to function. Let's say you put on 5 lb of muscle – you'll burn through an additional 150 calories a day just to fuel it. Fat, meanwhile, doesn't require any calories to function. It just sits there. It's doing nothing. It isn't responsible for any bodily functions, such as strength and movement. Its sole purpose is to provide stored energy.

CARBS FOR BURN MODE

One of the biggest misconceptions about nutrition is that you need to be on a high-protein plan if you want to go into calorie deficit and burn fat and lose weight. In my opinion, deficit means deficit – get there with a healthy, balanced macro breakdown. It's fine to monitor yourself and see how you feel on a daily basis. If you have a lack of energy, add more carbohydrates and essential fats. From my experience, you should be eating more carbohydrates. Most people will say the opposite, but I don't care. This is the approach that has got results for my clients.

If you feel as though the body is breaking down and not repairing, feel free to add more protein. We all have different tastes and preferences; listen to your body and give it what it needs. Never feel guilty and stay in control. For instance, your macro breakdown could be 90 per cent carbohydrates and 10 per cent protein and fat, but if you're still in deficit – below your metabolic calorie requirement – your body still has to find an energy source such as fat. That will allow you to reduce your body-fat percentage.

You need more energy to complete your workouts when you're in burn mode. I like sessions to be longer and steadier with no rest phases to maintain a healthy and sustained fuel burn. How are you supposed to do those workouts when your energy levels are depleted and your concentration is compromised through a lack of carbs? It's far more beneficial to get into deficit – which will get you into burn mode – through more output (activity) than through limiting your input (reducing calories). You have to be a little bit careful, though, because if you go too far into calorie deficit, you can be compromised and go catabolic, which is when the body starts burning muscle tissue as energy (thus destroying your metabolism). You need to get that mix just right, where it's teetering just on the edge.

I always feel that when I'm burning fat as energy, my body feels the most efficient. You can always sense when your body switches into burn mode.

BE FLEXIBLE

Within your themes, be aware of how many calories you require that day. Always adjust to maintain your performance. Whether I was at the studio or on location with Daniel, I would monitor what he was being asked to do that day. If he was filming a stunt scene, I would add calories, and if it was a dialogue day and he wasn't going to be that active, I would alter the macros and the calories (without ever depriving him). When I was working with Chris Evans in preparation for *Captain America*, he was having 2,500–3,000 calories a day, but on a heavy lifting day I would normally add 500 more protein calories to aid repair.

While I am in a privileged position as I work with professional chefs to ensure my clients' nutrition is just right, you could also consider what you might need on any given day. I think of this as 'engineered nutrition', because you're constantly adjusting your intake to tailor it to you and your day.

Most people are in the habit of eating three large meals a day, which can make you feel bloated and lethargic. It also takes the body longer to digest the food. That's why I encourage actors, and now you, to eat more often but have smaller meals – it's like having six brunches a day.

With a shorter break between meals, you spend less time thinking about when you're going to eat next, and you're also less likely to reach for the unhealthy snacks. Mentally, it's great knowing that you're going to be eating again soon. The boost in energy and the psychological benefits from eating six small meals a day are noticeable.

I'm a realist, and I appreciate that it's going to be harder for you than for an actor who has a chef on hand to prepare fast and efficient meals for them, but I still think six brunches a day is achievable for anyone. Anything in life is possible if you want to do it, but you will have to get organized. The body loves patterns and routines, so once you have devised one – eating every two or three hours with this six-brunches-a-day plan – it creates a good habit.

FOR GOOD GUT HEALTH, DON'T EAT TOO CLEAN

Most mornings on the set of *No Time to Die*, Daniel and I would have a balanced breakfast of rye toast, poached eggs, avocado, kale and sauerkraut. Quite a contrast from the on-set breakfast I saw him eating when I met him for the first time, when he emerged from a trailer eating a bacon sandwich.

As a natural probiotic, the sauerkraut helped to improve his gut health. You can put the best food into your body, but if you haven't got good gut health – with efficient breakdown, absorption and distribution – then it's pointless. You won't be getting the best performance from your high-quality food. In my experience, you'll know you have good gut health – as well as good health – if you have energy and you're sleeping well, which is always a sign that everything is in balance.

People always talk about eating clean, and cutting out all processed foods. In my view, you don't want to be too clean because then you potentially compromise what is happening in your gut. If you eat too clean, and you don't mix your food groups, your body may possibly decide it no longer needs certain bacteria in the gut and stops producing them. I work on the theory that if you don't use it, you lose it, so always ensure your body is always doing what it is designed to do. In addition to sauerkraut, I can recommend kefir, a fermented yoghurt, which provides good gut health. Any food that is rich in probiotics, or even a live supplement source, is going to help you to maintain a healthy gut.

CREATING AN ANTI-INFLAMMATORY STATE

When you're training hard, you want to put your body into an anti-inflammatory state, which is why I encourage actors to have daily shots of turmeric or ginger. Turmeric and ginger are great natural anti-inflammatories and help the body to be less toxic and inflamed.

To get adaptation, you have to damage your body through working out. Your body responds by adapting and strengthening itself but, as part of that process, you're inevitably going to get inflammation without you even realizing it. But if you can put yourself into an anti-inflammatory state by drinking a daily shot of turmeric or having a cup of turmeric tea, you're going to be reducing that inflammation. I also love wheatgrass shots for their energy-providing, natural medicinal feel, as well as lemon and ginger shots to boost the immune system.

ANTI-INFLAMMATORY TURMERIC TONIC

Try this anti-inflammatory turmeric tonic, using a recipe created by chef Sarah Sugden.

You'll need:

> 6 pieces of fresh turmeric root, each piece roughly an
>   inch long
> 3 pieces of fresh ginger root
> Juice from 2 lemons or oranges
> 2 tablespoons of manuka or raw honey
> 3 pinches of ground black pepper

Wash or scrub away any dirt on the turmeric and ginger roots, but keep the skin on both. Place all the ingredients in a high-speed blender and blend until smooth. Strain through a nut-milk bag or fine sieve. You can have it straight up as a powerful shot or prepare a warming tea by adding three-quarters of a tablespoon to a mug of boiled water. For a refreshing and hydrating tonic, you can add it to sparkling water, ice and fresh mint leaves. For a metabolic boost, add a pinch of cayenne, while a pinch of cinnamon will improve blood flow and circulation.

Eating triggers all sorts of emotional and chemical reactions in terms of how the food tastes, smells and also looks. That's why food presentation is so important, because if it looks good it'll make you feel good. Food doesn't have to be bland or boring; if meals look appetizing on your plate, it'll encourage you to have a healthy relationship with food. As the saying goes, you eat with your eyes.

PRE- AND POST-PERFORMANCE BOOSTS

Daniel Craig and I liked to have an espresso before working out and I recommend that you do the same (if you like coffee). I find that an espresso is the best possible stimulation before you start training, as you're getting a caffeine hit and it also tastes and smells great. It's the ideal way to signal to yourself and your senses that you're about to work out. Having an espresso is even better before exercising with a friend, as a pre-workout coffee is a good way to integrate some social activity into your programme, and also gives you time to discuss the session you're about to do.

There are also zero calories in an espresso, so I believe it's much better for you than sports or energy drinks, which are packed full of refined sugar. If you like to have sugary drinks before training because that works for you, that's fine, but there are undoubtedly effects on your health from consuming all that sugar, so you could consider switching to coffee.

After a workout at Pinewood Studios, Daniel and I would have a plant-based, post-workout performance shake – made with nut milk, protein and greens – as we walked from the gym to prepare for work. In my view, that shake would always set the tone for the day on set, as Daniel would be thinking about nutrition as a performance enhancer rather than something to be consumed in a social setting.

DANIEL'S POST-PERFORMANCE SHAKE

What you'll need for Daniel's *No Time to Die* performance shake, using Sarah Sugden's recipe:

    1 banana
    1 scoop of plant-based protein powder (pea/brown rice protein)
    2 large handfuls of fresh spinach
    1 cup of plant-based milk (oat, almond, hemp)
    1 tablespoon each of hemp seeds, goji berries and chia seeds
    1 teaspoon of organic maca root powder
    A dash of cinnamon

This is very easy to make – just blend all the ingredients together with a small handful of ice in a high-speed blender.

To lower the carbohydrate content, omit the banana or just use half (keep a zip-locked bag of peeled banana pieces in the freezer to have them at the ready). If you prefer a less creamy drink, substitute the plant milk for coconut water. When choosing a plant protein powder, look for one with pure and simple ingredients. If you prefer a sweeter taste, go for one with stevia or vanilla. For an extra layer of nutrition, add a scoop of your favourite super-greens blend, which might contain wheatgrass, spirulina and barley grass.

Timing is crucial. Where possible, and if your programme dictates, you should try to consume the shake within twenty to thirty minutes after completing a workout, as that's when the body is most receptive to refuelling. During that post-workout window, cells in your body are actively looking to receive and store nutritional energy for use later. I like to think your energy today is a reflection of what you stored yesterday.

I prefer plant-based proteins, such as split pea and hemp, as they have fewer chemicals and feel better for the gut. I believe they are easier to break down and distribute. It feels a lot more natural and nourishing. You're never just refuelling the body; you're also refuelling your mind. Those shakes – which were always pre-prepared and kept in the fridge in the gym – became an important part of our morning ritual.

FIND YOUR OWN WAY

The body is going to tell you what it wants. If you become more attuned to what's happening within it, you will start to become able to read those signals more readily. The body has a funny way of telling you when it needs something upon which it's reliant. That could be caffeine, sugar, protein, carbohydrates or, most importantly, water. I believe that you need to learn not to be so reactive to these signals, but to be more preventative. If you know that your energy levels generally start to dip at 11 a.m., take preventative action by having something to eat or drink half an hour before.

As we start out on our fitness journeys, we often prioritize the output and what we plan to do, when in actual fact our focus should be on our input and recovery. What you put into your body determines what you get out of it. As you feel yourself making progress, you can start asking yourself what it will take to look and feel even fitter. You naturally begin to tell yourself to cut down on refined sugars and start implementing the other little everyday adjustments you can make to your nutrition plan. Small changes will always turn into big gains.

Ultimately, you need to discover what works for you. It's important that you cultivate your own relationship with nutrition. Pick and choose elements of what I've advised here, but please feel free to follow your own path as it's best to find a way that's sustainable for you. In my experience, people are much more compliant when they are making their own decisions; they're then far more likely to make healthy choices.

In the end, the nutritional aspect of fitness is very simple. It's about motivation and finding what suits you, which can be sustained over the long term, and it's also about what you enjoy and what's going to make you happy.

14 | STAYING HYDRATED

Water is the source of life. It's the biggest healer and the best energy provider. It's therefore no surprise that it's incredibly important to make sure that you are properly hydrated – not just while you're exercising, but before and after too. Water regulates pretty much everything in your body, from your temperature to the functioning of your organs, to delivering nutrients to the cells in your body.

Of course, while water is the purest way to hydrate, milk, tea, coffee and soft drinks are all made up of over 85 per cent water and can form part of your total fluid intake. I'm very relaxed about my clients drinking coffee and having an occasional glass of wine, just so long as they are also drinking enough water. Stay hydrated but go ahead and have an espresso or a glass of something if you feel like one. Find the right balance between being hydrated and stimulated. If you are a big coffee drinker, try to copy the Italians who have a glass of water alongside an espresso. That water helps to cleanse your palate so you can taste the coffee; it also prevents you from becoming dehydrated.

One great habit to get into is to drink a glass of water as soon as you get up. I also recommend having some water just before you go to bed, but maybe not too much as you don't want to be waking up in the middle of the night.

You should always have water with you, and try to keep drinking throughout the day. You shouldn't be drinking so much

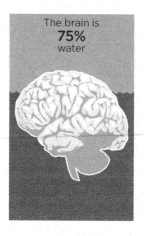
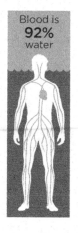
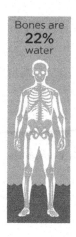
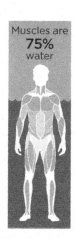

The brain is **75%** water

Blood is **92%** water

Bones are **22%** water

Muscles are **75%** water

water in one go that it's sloshing around inside you, as that can affect digestion; instead sip small amounts all day. If you're not used to drinking a healthy amount of water, you need to get your body used to being hydrated, so slowly build up the amount you're taking in. You will feel and see the difference in no time: healthier skin, brighter eyes and better overall wellbeing.

If you like, you can add hydration tablets to your water, which contain electrolytes and key minerals. This becomes more important in a hot and humid environment, or when you're doing a long and arduous training day when the body is sweating more than normal.

While my clients understand the importance of hydrating while training with me, I like them to sip between exercises but not to have extended water breaks. It's better to avoid spending a couple of minutes hanging out at the water fountain in the gym. You might be hydrating, but you're losing intensity and your heart rate is dropping, and you're also wasting valuable gym time.

The body's signal for thirst – which it sends up the spinal cord to the brain – is very similar to the signal for hunger. If you think you can sense the signal for hunger, it's possible that your brain is actually trying to tell you that you're thirsty and you've misinterpreted it as a hunger pang. Have a glass of water first and see if that feeling disappears. Maybe you're not even hungry at all.

IT'S ALL IN THE PREP

Two weeks before Jake Gyllenhaal arrived in the Sahara to shoot *Prince of Persia*, I asked him to start increasing the amount of water he was drinking and to boost his electrolytes. If you've got a big event or a trip coming up in a hot country, and you know you're going to be working in oppressive conditions, you should start your hydration protocols a fortnight in advance. Once you're there, you can't expect an instant fix, and if you do feel dehydrated, it's already too late and it's very tough to sort out your hydration levels.

That's why preparation really is key to giving you the best chance of avoiding dehydration. You have to give your body the time to adjust to drinking more water, and also the time to absorb the salts and minerals from any supplements you're taking. You're allowing your body to store what it needs so it can use it later.

CONCLUSION

Having read this book and engaged with the workouts and routines, my hope is that you now find yourself in a similar position to many of my clients. I'm confident that Daniel Craig learned so much from the process of training for the role of James Bond – discovering what he liked and didn't like in terms of workouts and routines, and the occasional thing that I'm sure he'll be happy to never do again! I also believe that he will continue to maintain good fitness with so many tried-and-tested techniques now part of his exercise repertoire, and view his Bond training years as a fitness toolbox to dip into. I hope you will use this book in a similar way.

I'm sure there are certain elements of prepping for Bond that Daniel's never going to let go. Now he's finished with the character, he could in theory put some of the specific fitness stuff aside and just do what he enjoys, but I don't think that's in his mentality. I imagine that those strong elements of the programme are probably ingrained to some degree – from the training and the recovery to the nutrition – and that fitness and wellbeing are now a natural part of his day, even when he's not working. I like to think that Daniel will always have that intelligent fitness mindset.

As well as providing a solid insight into what it takes to reboot your body, using my methods that have turned some of the world's leading screen actors into athletes, most of all I hope that this book has inspired you. I would encourage you to try as many workouts in the book as you feel able to, and to use the tips and the advice to help you to achieve your own goals.

Perhaps you'll need different inspiration at different times, depending on how you're feeling and where you're at in your fitness journey. Maybe today you're more in the mood for a Léa Seydoux workout and tomorrow you'll want to train like Blake Lively, or perhaps you find yourself alternating between Chris Pratt's workout and the sessions that I created for John Boyega. Mix and match as you please. This should be a book that you can return to time and again, when you're looking for guidance and technical tips on how to do certain exercises, but also when you're in need of some motivation.

After many years of working in the industry and achieving some incredible body transformations, my belief in performance over aesthetic is stronger than ever. As I have said throughout this book, fitness is a feeling – it's about feeling that your body is working with you, rather than against you, that you're ageing well and not letting your physical health fall by the wayside. I feel that an intelligent approach to fitness is key to a healthier life. We need to train in a way that's fun, exhilarating and interesting. We need to understand how our body works, to know when to push it and when to let it recover.

Don't give yourself a hard time if the results aren't immediate. Be kind to yourself, put the work in and the positive changes will follow. I think one of the most important messages in this book is that you need to find what works for you. This is not only the most sustainable approach to lifelong fitness, but it's also the most intelligent. Train like a child, listen to your body and, above all, enjoy it!

ACKNOWLEDGEMENTS

Everyone that I've ever worked with over the years has contributed to this book in some way. The actors wouldn't have known it at the time, but they trained me just as much as I trained them. I'm particularly grateful to Daniel Craig for writing the foreword for this book, and for encouraging me to pursue this project in the first place. Photographer Greg Williams is a genius, and very generously opened up his Bond archive of behind-the-scenes shots for the photo section of this book, as well as taking the cover photo of me. Many thanks to Mark Hodgkinson for helping me shape the words, and to Jo Stansall, Saskia Angenent and the rest of the team at Michael O'Mara Books for their encouragement and support. I'm also thankful to Nick Walters, David Luxton and Rebecca Winfield at David Luxton Associates for their energy and enthusiasm throughout this project.

PICTURE CREDITS

PLATE SECTION 1

Most of the photos: author's own

Additional sources:

© Greg Williams: 2 (above, below); 3 (above). © Shutterstock: 3 (below) Jay Maidment / Eon / Danjaq / Sony / Kobal / Shutterstock. © Alamy: 4 (below) Lucasfilm / Picturelux / The Hollywood Archive / Alamy; 8 (below) Lucasfilm / © Walt Disney Studios / Everett Collection / Alamy.

PLATE SECTION 2

Most of the photos: author's own

Additional sources:

© Greg Williams: 1; 2 (above, below); 3; 5 (above, below); 6(above, below); 8 (above)

INDEX